PROBLEMS IN
MEDICAL MICROBIOLOGY

Problems in
Medical Microbiology

JOHN HOLTON
BSc MB ChB PhD MRCPath
Department of Medical Microbiology
University College London Medical School

NICOLA BRINK
MB CHB MMed (Virol) MRCPath
Division of Virology
Department of Medical Microbiology
University College London Medical School

PETER CHIODINI
BSc MBBS PhD FRCP
Department of Clinical Parasitology
The Hospital for Tropical Diseases
London

RICHARD BENDALL
BSc MBBS MRCP MRCPath DTMott
Department of Clinical Parasitology
The Hospital for Tropical Diseases
London

b

Blackwell
Science

© 1995 by
Blackwell Science Ltd
Editorial Offices:
Osney Mead, Oxford OX2 0EL
25 John Street, London WC1N 2BL
23 Ainslie Place, Edinburgh EH3 6AJ
238 Main Street, Cambridge
    Massachusetts 02142, USA
54 University Street, Carlton
    Victoria 3053, Australia

Other Editorial Offices:
Arnette Blackwell SA
  1, rue de Lille, 75007 Paris
  France

Blackwell Wissenschafts-Verlag GmbH
  Kurfürstendamm 57
  10707 Berlin, Germany
  Feldgasse 13, A-1238 Wien
  Austria

First published 1995

Set by Excel Typesetters Company, Hong Kong
Printed and bound in Italy by G. Canale, SpA,
Turin.

distributors

Marston Book Services Ltd
PO Box 87
Oxford OX2 0DT
(*Orders*: Tel: 01865 791155
         Fax: 01865 791927
         Telex: 837515)

North America
Blackwell Science, Inc.
238 Main Street
Cambridge, MA 02142
(*Orders*: Tel: 800 215-1000
           617 876-7000
       Fax: 617 492-5263)

Australia
Blackwell Science Pty Ltd
54 University Street
Carlton, Victoria 3053
(*Orders*: Tel: 03 347-0300
           03 349-3016)

A catalogue record for this title
is available from the British Library

ISBN 0-632-03834-9 (BSL)
ISBN 0-632-03836-5 (Four Dragons)

Library of Congress
Cataloging-in-Publication Data

Problems in medical microbiology/ John Holton
. . . [et al.].
        p.   cm.
    Includes bibliographical references.
    ISBN 0-632-03834-9
    1. Medical microbiology—Examinations,
    questions, etc.
  1. Holton, John, MRCPath.
    [DNLM: 1. Microbiology—problems.
    2. Bacterial Infections—diagnosis—problems.
    3. Bacterial Infections—drug therapy—problems.
    4. Virus Diseases—diagnosis—problems.
    5. Virus Diseases—drug therapy—problems.
    6. Parasitology—problems.   QW 18 P962 1995]
    QR46.P85   1995
    616'.01'076—dc20
    DNLM/DLC for Library of Congress
                                        94-38954
                                             CIP

Contents

Preface

Medical education in the UK has traditionally been based on systematic teaching. However, recent recommendations by the General Medical Council in the UK have emphasized the need for the establishment of a core of factual knowledge, supplemented by a problem-orientated approach to medical education, which allows the student to gain experience in clinical problem solving. In line with these changes, this book attempts to provide the student with practice in interpreting laboratory results within the context of a clinical microbiological problem. This book is based upon part of the clinical microbiology course given at University College London Medical School.

Acknowledgements

We would like to thank our colleagues for providing some of the photographs in this book: Dr G L Ridgway; Dr G M Scott; Mr A Cremer of the Clinical Microbiology Department, UCL Hospitals, London; Dr I R Ferguson of Hereford PHL County Hospital, Hereford.

Figure 53.1, courtesy of Dr J Fox; Fig. 53.2, courtesy of E M Briggs; Fig. 55.1, courtesy of Professor D Crawford; Fig. 56.1, reproduced with permission from *The Practitioner* 1988, **232**. 1988; Fig. 57.1, reproduced with permission from *Public Health Virology —12 reports* (1986), Mortimer P (ed.); Fig. 57.2, courtesy of Professor J Pattison; Fig. 58.1, courtesy of Professor J Pattison; Fig. 59.1, reproduced from Reid D, Grist N R & Pinkerton I W, *Infections in Current Medical Practice*; Fig. 60.2, courtesy of E M Briggs; Fig. 63.1, courtesy of J C Waite; Fig. 64.1, courtesy of E M Briggs; Fig. 65.1, courtesy of J C Waite; Fig. 66.1 courtesy of Professor R Tedder; Fig. 66.2, courtesy of E M Briggs; Fig. 67.1, courtesy of J D Fox; Fig. 70.1, reproduced from Mindel A & Adler M W (1984), *Genital Herpes Lecture Kit* Gower Medical Publishing Ltd., for the Wellcome Foundation Ltd., London.

Bacteria and Fungi

A 30-year-old man had a cough productive of rusty-coloured sputum. He had a pleuritic chest pain and was pyrexial (39°C) and short of breath. He had diminished movements over the right side of his chest and on auscultation he was noted to have crepitations. There was increased fremitus and percussion was dull over his right chest posteriorly. His chest X-ray revealed a homogeneous opacity over part of his lung field. His white blood count was 25 × 10⁹/l with 70% polymorphonuclear leucocytes.

A sputum sample was taken, and a Gram stain performed. Figure 1.1 shows a Gram stain of the sputum sample and the blood agar plate (Fig. 1.2) shows the results of culture of the sputum.

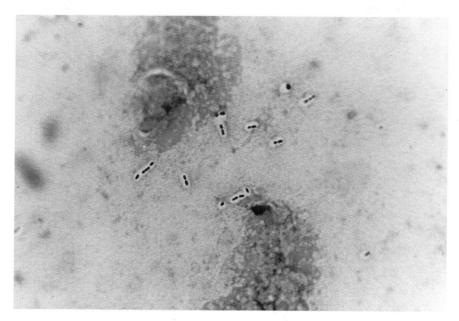

Fig. 1.1

1

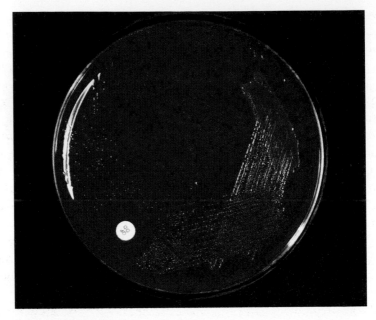

Fig. 1.2 OPT, optochin.

Questions
1 What is the identity of the organism?
2 From what clinical illness is the patient suffering?
3 What other specimens would have been useful in making the diagnosis and how would they have been processed?
4 How should the patient be managed?
5 Which one of the following antimicrobial agents would be appropriate in the treatment of this patient:
   (a) benzylpenicillin?
   (b) flucloxacillin?
   (c) metronidazole?
   (d) mebendazole?

Answers

1 The organism is identified as *Streptococcus pneumoniae* because of the following attributes.

(a) It is a Gram-positive coccus (Fig. 1.1). The organisms are typically in pairs and the clear, unstained zone around the organisms shows that a large capsule is present. Some patients are more prone to becoming infected with capsulate organisms such as *S. pneumoniae*, for example, those who have undergone splenectomy. Such patients should be on long-term prophylactic oral penicillin (phenoxymethyl penicillin, penicillin V) and if possible should have been given pneumococcal vaccine (e.g. pneumovax II) prior to splenectomy. Pneumococcal vaccine can also prevent severe pneumococcal disease in some groups of otherwise healthy individuals.

(b) It is an α-haemolytic streptococcus (sometimes called viridans streptococcus because of the area of greening around the colonies, caused by partial haemolysis of the blood; Fig. 1.2). Alpha-haemolytic streptococci are found mainly in the oropharynx where they form part of the normal flora. There are many different named species of viridans streptococci; one is a cause of dental caries and others are the principal cause of endocarditis (e.g. *S. sanguis*). The other main groups of streptococci are β-haemolytic streptococci, enterococci and anaerobic streptococci.

(c) The growth is inhibited by optochin (Fig. 1.2). Of all the viridans streptococci, only *S. pneumoniae* is inhibited by optochin. Therefore, this is used as a quick means of identification in the laboratory.

2 A patient who presents with purulent sputum, a high temperature, pleuritic chest pain, dyspnoea and neutrophilia with localized signs in the chest accompanied by a lobar opacity on a chest X-ray is suffering from lobar pneumonia – the principal cause of which is *S. pneumoniae*. *S. pneumoniae* is also a cause of conjunctivitis, otitis media and sinusitis, empyema, infective episodes in chronic bronchitis, meningitis and septicaemia. The organisms associated with chronic bronchitis are often non-capsulate, whereas serious invasive disease is often caused by capsulate strains, as in this case.

3 A patient whom you suspect of having pneumonia should have a blood culture taken in addition to a sputum specimen. A urine specimen may also be useful, as the capsule material of *S. pneumoniae* is excreted into the urine and can be detected by a rapid latex agglutination test. In the

1 laboratory the organism isolated from the specimens can be identified and its sensitivity to antibiotics determined. If it is clinically appropriate, the capsular type of the infecting strain of *S. pneumoniae* can be determined.

4 The patient should be given parenteral benzylpenicillin. Depending upon the clinical severity, oral amoxycillin would be an alternative choice.

Penicillin-resistant pneumococci and pneumococci resistant to a range of antibiotics are being isolated more frequently. Alternative antibiotics that may be of use are erythromycin, cotrimoxazole, cefuroxime, chloramphenicol and tetracycline, depending upon the sensitivities. The patient may also require physiotherapy or ventilation support.

5 (a) Benzylpenicillin is the appropriate antibiotic.

(b) Flucloxacillin is also a β-lactam but is used specifically for infections caused by benzylpenicillin-resistant *Staphylococcus aureus*.

(c) Metronidazole is an antibiotic used to treat infections caused by anaerobes, pseudomembranous colitis and infections caused by *Trichomonas vaginalis* and *Giardia lamblia*.

(d) Mebendazole is an antibiotic that is used to treat a number of helminth infections such as threadworm (*Enterobius*) and hookworm (*Ancylostoma*).

References

Carbon C & Leophonte P (1993) Management of community-acquired pneumonia. *J. Antimicrob. Chemother.* **32**, 1–3.

Fass RJ (1993) Aetiology and treatment of community-acquired pneumonia in adults. *J. Antimicrob. Chemother.* **32** (Suppl. A), 17–27.

An obese 45-year-old female was admitted to an intensive care unit (ICU) **2**
following a road traffic accident, where she was placed on a ventilator. An
initial chest X-ray was reported as normal. Five days after admission to
the ICU the patient's condition deteriorated. She developed an elevated
temperature, a neutrophilia and signs of bilateral basal consolidation in
the chest. Specimens of a tracheal aspirate were collected for microscopy
(Fig. 2.1) and culture, along with a blood culture, from which an organism
identical to the one in the tracheal aspirate was isolated.

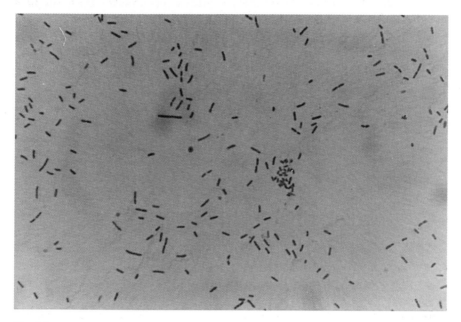

Fig. 2.1

Questions
1 Which bacteria typically cause chest infections under these clinical circumstances? Which antibiotic would you choose to treat the patient
  with?
2 Describe the factors leading to the development of pneumonia in ventilated patients.

2 Answers

1 Clinically this is a case of nosocomially acquired, ventilator-associated pneumonia. The organisms most frequently responsible for pneumonia under these conditions are Gram-negative bacilli, either coliforms (e.g. *Escherichia, Klebsiella, Enterobacter, Serratia*) or pseudomonads (e.g. *Pseudomonas aeruginosa*). Because many of these organisms are part of the environmental flora of ICUs and hospitals in general, they are often multi-antibiotic-resistant. The antibiotic groups most frequently used in these circumstances are aminoglycosides (e.g. gentamicin), β-lactams (e.g. cefuroxime, ceftazidime, imipenem) or quinolones (e.g. ciprofloxacin). The antibiotic chosen would depend upon the results of the *in vitro* sensitivity testing from the microbiology laboratory.

Antibiotic resistance is due to: (a) inactivation of antibiotics by modification or destruction, brought about by plasmid or chromosomally coded enzymes; (b) a change in the permeability of the bacterial cell wall to antibiotics caused by chromosomal mutations; or (c) an alteration of the target. Aminoglycosides are modified by several different enzymes (acetyltransferases, phosphotransferases, adenyltransferases) and the resistant phenotype of the organism depends upon which plasmid-coded enzyme the organism possesses. Some strains of bacteria may be resistant to all aminoglycosides except gentamicin (6′ acetyltransferase) or resistant to gentamicin yet sensitive to amikacin(2″ adenyltransferase). Resistance to fluoroquinolones is caused by chromosomal mutations which alter the target of the antibiotic−deoxyribonucleic acid (DNA) gyrase. Resistance to β-lactams is mediated by enzymes that hydrolyse the antibiotic (β-lactamases) and they can be coded for by plasmids (e.g. TEM-1) or the chromosome. TEM-1 codes for β-lactamases that hydrolyse broad-spectrum penicillins (e.g. ampicillin). Recently detected plasmid-coded β-lactamases, derived by mutations of TEM-1, can hydrolyse monobactams (e.g. aztreonam). Inducible chromosomally mediated β-lactamases are produced by several coliforms or pseudomonads and mutation in the *amp* C locus can lead to constitutive production of the β-lactamases (e.g. in *Enterobacter cloacae*) which have an extended spectrum of activity against cephamycins, monobactams and antipseudomonal penicillins. Beta-lactamases hydrolysing carbapenems (e.g. imipenem) have been detected in *Stenotrophomonas*.

2 A great deal of evidence points to the stomach as a reservoir for organisms causing ventilator-associated pneumonia. Overgrowth of bacteria

in the stomach may occur because of gastric motility disorders (e.g. gastroduodenal reflux) or because the patient has been given H$_2$-receptor antagonists in an attempt to reduce stress-related ulceration of the stomach. Regurgitation of stomach contents in a ventilated patient can then lead to aspiration into the lungs to initiate a pneumonia, despite the presence of an endotracheal tube. Colonization of the oropharynx by exogenously acquired microflora has been suggested as an alternative source of infection.

References

Inglis TJJ, Sherratt M, Sproat LJ, Gibson JS & Hawkey PM (1993) Gastroduodenal dysfunction and bacterial colonisation of the ventilated lung. *Lancet* **341**, 911–913.

Wenzel RP (1989) Hospital-acquired pneumonia: overview of the current state of the art for prevention and control. *Eur. J. Clin. Microbiol. Infect. Dis.* **8**, 56–60.

3 A 31-year-old homosexual male was admitted to hospital complaining of shortness of breath and generalized chest discomfort. A chest X-ray revealed diffuse bilateral opacities and a blood gas analysis demonstrated a Pao_2 of 8.0 kPa.

A bronchoalveolar lavage was performed and sent to the laboratory for microscopy (Fig. 3.1) and culture.

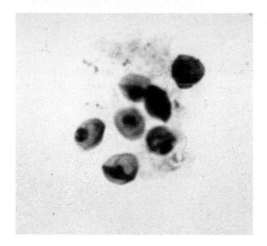

Fig. 3.1

Questions

1 What is the clinical diagnosis?
2 What microscopic investigation was performed and what does it show?
3 How should the patient be managed?

1 Clinically the patient is likely to have pneumonia caused by *Pneumocystis carinii* (PCP) which is the predominant respiratory illness in patients with acquired immune deficiency syndrome (AIDS). This organism, which is probably a fungus, is believed to be acquired at a young age and reactivates with waning immunity; the organism multiplies within the lungs and causes symptoms. There is some evidence for a seasonal prevalence of pneumonia caused by PCP, which would support acquisition of the organism as an adult. PCP typically presents with shortness of breath, usually in the absence of purulent sputum or pleuritic pain, although the patient may have a cough. Patients are frequently pyrexial. There is no typical X-ray appearance in patients with PCP as they may have bilateral hilar opacities, nodular opacities or even a normal chest X-ray. Computerised tomography (CT) and gallium-67 scans of the lungs may pick up abnormalities not seen on a plain X-ray. Arterial blood gas analysis shows hypoxaemia due to diminished diffusion of oxygen into the blood and hypocapnia due to tachypnoea. Exercise can cause further desaturation of the blood. An induced sputum or bronchoalveolar lavage specimen should be sent to the laboratory for detection of PCP and routine culture.

2 PCP can be detected in the sputum or lavage specimen by staining with methenamine silver stain, where the typical cysts can be seen, as shown in Fig. 3.1. Culture for PCP is not part of the routine work-up for this pathogen, although the specimen should be cultured for coexisting bacterial pathogens. PCP may also be detected by use of the polymerase chain reaction.

3 The treatment of choice is high-dose co-trimoxazole.
   Many patients with AIDS have hypersensitivity reactions to sulphonamides and under these circumstances alternative treatments for PCP are: aerosolized or parenteral pentamidine; dapsone and trimethoprim, primaquine and clindamycin or atovaquone. After an attack of PCP the patient must be kept on a prophylactic regimen. Even though a patient may have reacted adversely to co-trimoxazole in treatment doses, the use of co-trimoxazole for prophylaxis may be free of side-effects. Other maintenance regimens that can be used are pentamidine, dapsone or Fansidar.

3 References

Clumeck N, Hermans P & DeWit S (1988) Current problems in the management of AIDS patients. *Eur. J. Clin. Microbiol. Infect. Dis.* **7**, 2–10.

Millar AB & Hind CRK (1991) Aids and the lung. *Hosp. Update* **17**, 177–190.

A previously healthy 50-year-old patient who smoked heavily was admitted to hospital with a diagnosis of pneumonia shortly after returning from holiday abroad. The patient had received a 3-day course of amoxycillin from his general practitioner, with no effect on the clinical condition. A chest X-ray was performed (Fig. 4.1). The patient was not producing sputum to be cultured. A blood culture was taken which did not grow anything after 48h of incubation. Whilst in hospital, the patient became confused and laboratory tests indicated a serum sodium of 120mmol/l and an elevated creatinine level.

4

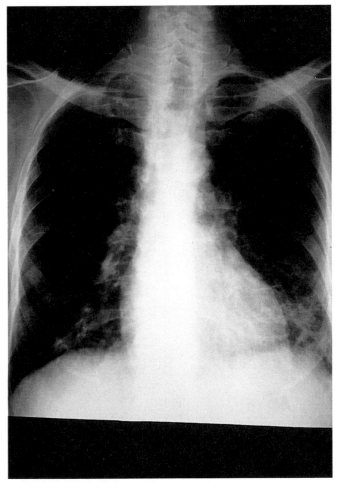

Fig. 4.1

4 Questions

1 What is your clinical diagnosis and how would you confirm it?
2 Which antibiotic should the patient be given?
3 What public health measures have to be considered?

1 The patient is unlikely to have pneumococcal pneumonia because he was not producing any sputum and the chest X-ray shows a diffuse bilateral basal opacity rather than the lobar opacity seen in pneumococcal pneumonia. The patient has not responded to amoxycillin, which would have been expected with pneumococcal pneumonia, unless the patient had been infected with a penicillin-resistant strain. Currently, the prevalence of penicillin resistance in *Streptococcus pneumoniae* is low, although some countries do have high prevalence rates, for example, Spain. It is therefore important to have established an exact geographical history. These facts, taken together with the sex, age, smoking history and biochemical evidence of renal involvement, suggest an atypical pneumonia, for example, legionnaires' disease.

Legionellae are fastidious organisms with a Gram-negative type of cell-wall structure that are widespread in environmental water sources and colonize institutional, hotel and domestic water supplies. The bacteria are maintained intracellularly in various species of amoeba found in water. Humans become infected by breathing in aerosols of contaminated water from cooling towers and air-conditioning systems. Person-to-person transmission has not been reported. Hospital water supplies may also be contaminated with *Legionella* and nosocomial outbreaks of legionnaires' disease have been reported. The amount of *Legionella* in water supplies can be minimized by periodic hyperchlorination or boosting the water temperature in order to kill the organism.

Sputum (if available) or bronchoalveolar lavage specimens, along with serum and urine, should be sent to the laboratory. *L. pneumophila* can be cultured on selective media (buffered charcoal–yeast extract agar); it takes 2–3 days to form colonies, although the organism cannot generally be demonstrated in the specimen using the Gram stain. Direct immunofluorescent stains can be used to detect *Legionella* in the respiratory specimen. An antibody response may be detected in the serum, but antibody levels may rise slowly and may not be detected for several weeks after the respiratory illness. *Legionella* antigen may be detected in the urine.

2 The treatment of choice for legionnaires' disease is erythromycin. The newer macrolides, for example, clarithromycin and azithromycin, are deserving of further study. If the patient does not respond, rifampicin should be given with the erythromycin. Successful therapy has also been reported with the use of quinolones (e.g. ciprofloxacin, ofloxacin),

4 although treatment failures have also been reported with quinolones given as a single agent.

3 Although sporadic cases of legionnaires' disease do occur, a single case admitted to hospital may be part of a larger outbreak. Outbreaks of legionnaires' disease acquired by holiday-makers who stayed at a particular hotel are known, and it is important for the clinician or microbiologist to liaise with the local consultant in communicable diseases about the possibility of an outbreak of legionnaires' disease.

References

Edelstein PH (1986) Control of *Legionella* in hospitals. *J. Hosp. Infect.* **8**, 109–115.
Winn WC (1988) Legionnaires disease: historical perspective. *Clin. Microbiol. Rev.* **1**, 60–81.

A 25-year-old female developed pharyngitis, a non-productive cough, 5
temperature, myalgia and an extensive maculopapular rash over the
period of a few days. On examination of the chest only occasional widespread crackles were heard and a chest X-ray was taken which showed
patchy shadows in both lung fields. A viral screen was negative, but it was
noted that a blood sample that had been collected for serological investigation and kept at 20°C had the effect shown in Fig. 5.1.

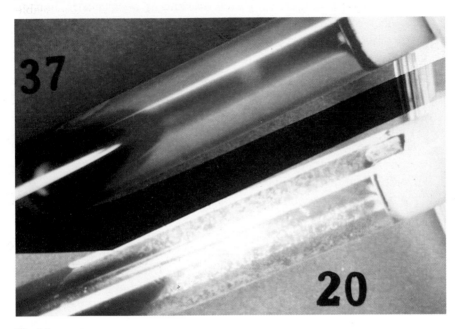

Fig. 5.1

Questions
1 What is your differential diagnosis for this patient's condition? What
   further information is required?
2 What is the explanation for the effect seen in Fig. 5.1?
3 How should the patient be managed?

5 Answers

1 The patient has pneumonia caused by *Mycoplasma pneumoniae*. The clinical presentation and radiological findings are that of an atypical pneumonia. This is a group of pneumonias that each present in a similar fashion with similar radiological findings but which are quite distinct from that of pneumococcal pneumonia. The bacteria that cause pneumonia presenting in this fashion are *Legionella pneumophila*, *Coxiella burnetii*, *Chlamydia psittaci*, *C. pneumoniae* and *M. pneumoniae*. There are a number of viruses that may present with a rash and pulmonary involvement, for example, adenovirus 7, varicella-zoster virus, measles virus, coxsackievirus A9, echovirus II, but in this patient there was no serological evidence of viral infection.

Both sporadic and epidemic cases of legionnaires' disease occur which can often be epidemiologically linked to an air-conditioning system as a source of infection. The patient is most likely to be a male who is a chronic smoker. Gastrointestinal symptoms are prominent and there is further evidence of systemic involvement with an altered mental state, renal involvement and hyponatraemia.

Psittacosis is a zoonosis. *C. psittaci* is shed in the excreta of birds and human infection may follow breathing in contaminated dust from these infected birds. A history of occupational or domestic contact with birds should be sought. Psittacosis presents with a sore throat, headache, myalgia, a non-productive cough and a rash resembling rose spots of enteric fever. Mental confusion may occur and hepatosplenomegaly may be present.

Pneumonia caused by *C. pneumoniae* is a milder pulmonary illness compared to the others. It too presents with a sore throat and cough, but hoarseness is a common feature, and a rash does not occur. Infection is contracted by inhalation of infected aerosols from another person or by indirect contact from contaminated objects.

C. burnetii causes a fever (Q fever) which is principally an occupational illness of farmers, veterinarians, dairy workers or laboratory workers. In this case the patient's occupation should be enquired into. *C. burnetii* is transmitted to humans by aerosols from infected cattle or sheep, or occasionally by drinking unpasteurized contaminated milk. The illness presents with a sudden onset of severe headache and a temperature. There may be pharyngitis, myalgia and a maculopapular rash and a characteristic bradycardia. Overt pulmonary involvement occurs in about 50% of patients, with dyspnoea and purulent sputum. Hepatomegaly may occur but jaundice is uncommon. Complications of infection can be aseptic meningitis, myocarditis, endocarditis, pancreatitis and orchitis.

2 Patients with pneumonia caused by *M. pneumoniae* may develop anti-I antibodies which cause agglutination of erythrocytes at 20°C (cold agglutinins). In this particular case the patient's own erythrocytes were agglutinated. This may lead to haemolytic anaemia developing. Other complications of pneumonia caused by *M. pneumoniae* are Stevens–Johnson syndrome, myringitis and myocarditis.

3 Patients should be treated with either tetracycline or erthromycin. Patients with Q fever should be treated with doxycycline. In cases of endocarditis caused by *C. burnetii*, patients should be treated with doxycycline and either co-trimoxazole or rifampicin. Patients with chlamydial infections (*C. pneumoniae, C. psittaci*) should be given doxycycline or erythromycin. Legionnaires' disease is treated with erythromycin, sometimes combined with rifampicin.

References

Cherry JD (1993) Anaemia and mucocutaneous lesions due to *M. pneumoniae* infections. *Clin. Infect. Dis.* **17** (Suppl. 1), 547–551.

Clyde WA (1993) Clinical overview of typical *M. pneumoniae* infections. *Clin. Infect. Dis.* **17** (Suppl. 1), 332–536.

Crosse BA (1990) Psittacosis: a clinical review. *J. Infect.* **21**, 251–259.

Grayson JT, Campbell LA, Kuo CC *et al.* (1990) A new respiratory tract pathogen: *Chlamydia pneumoniae* strain TWAR. *J. Infect. Dis.* **161**, 618–625.

6   An elderly male was seen on a domiciliary visit by his general practitioner who diagnosed influenza. This was confirmed by serology. On a return visit some days later the patient had deteriorated. He was admitted to hospital where he was found to have a high temperature and to be producing large amounts of purulent sputum. A chest X-ray was performed, which showed multiple abscesses, and sputum was sent for microscopy (Fig. 6.1) and culture. The organism was coagulase-positive and was inoculated onto a plate for the detection of DNase production (Fig. 6.2).

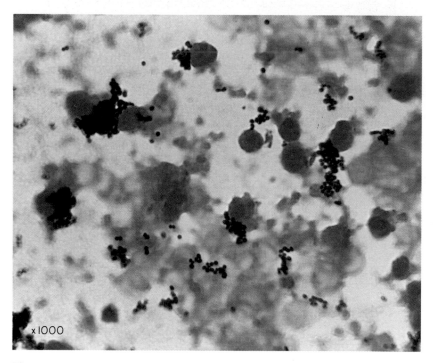

x1000

Fig. 6.1

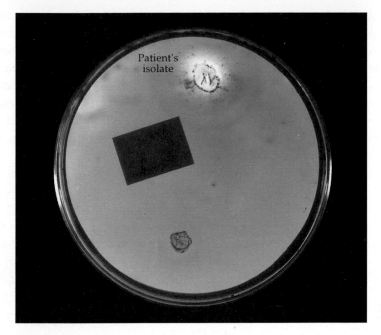

Fig. 6.2

Questions

1 What is the identity of the organism?
2 What further investigations may be necessary?
3 What is the appropriate antibiotic management of this patient?

6 Answers

1 *Staphylococcus aureus* is a likely cause of an acute onset of pneumonia following an attack of influenza. The organism commonly produces abscesses in the lungs. Pulmonary infection with *S. aureus* may also occur in patients who have cystic fibrosis. A Gram stain of the sputum demonstrates Gram-positive cocci in clusters—typical of staphylococcus. The production of coagulase and DNase identifies the organism as *S. aureus*. Many different species of coagulase-negative staphylococci exist and are found as part of the normal flora of the skin. The coagulase-negative staphylococci are typically causes of prosthetic valve endocarditis, infected joint prostheses and infected venous catheters.

The production of coagulase is determined by inoculation of the organism into plasma followed by incubation at 37°C. If the organism produces coagulase, then the plasma coagulates. The production of DNase is determined by inoculating the organism onto agar containing DNA. Hydrolysis of DNA by DNase (produced by *S. aureus*) is detected by flooding the plate with toluidine blue. A pink colour around the colony, as in Fig. 6.2, indicates the production of DNase.

2 *S. aureus* commonly produces pyogenic foci in many organs of the body following haematogenous spread. In this case, a patient who has had pneumonia with *S. aureus* is very likely to have had an associated bacteraemia and, if he does not respond, or relapses shortly after cessation of treatment, then one must consider a perinephric abscess, osteomyelitis or endocarditis and undertake further microbiological and radiological investigations—blood cultures, echocardiography, abdominal ultrasound and bone scans. Deep-seated chronic infections with *S. aureus* may also be diagnosed by detecting antibodies to secreted extracellular products of *S. aureus*, for example, anti-DNase antibodies.

3 The treatment must be guided by the sensitivity tests. Most *S. aureus* are sensitive to flucloxacillin and this is the most appropriate antibiotic. In the circumstances of this case it may be combined with fusidic acid or gentamicin.

Reference

Verhoef J & Verbrugh HA (1981) Host determinants in staphylococcal disease. *Annu. Rev. Med.* **32**, 107–122.

A nurse was admitted to hospital complaining of a persistent fever, general malaise and weight loss, over a period of 3 weeks. The patient was placed in isolation and a chest X-ray (Fig. 7.1), sputum culture and microscopy were performed (Figs 7.2 & 7.3).

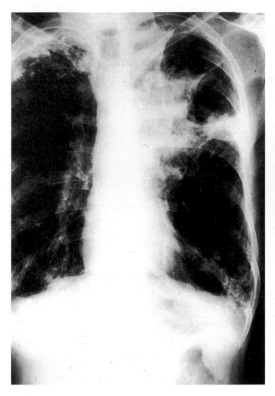

Fig. 7.1

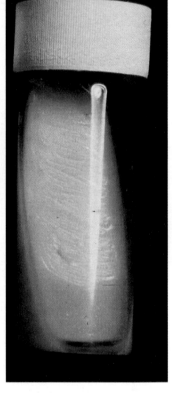

Fig. 7.2

7

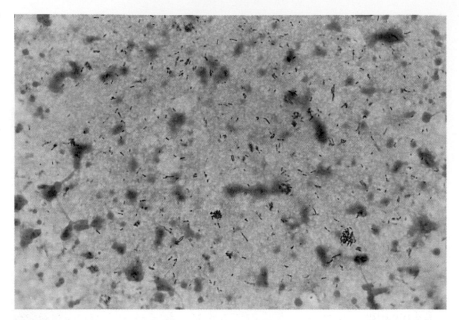

Fig. 7.3

Questions
1 What is the name of the stain (7.3) and culture medium (7.2) used?
2 What is the identity of the organism?
3 What other methods exist for the diagnosis of this organism?
4 How should this infection be managed?

1 The stain is called a Ziehl–Neelsen stain. Mycobacteria appear red using this stain (due to retention of carbolfuchsin after washing the slide with acid), whereas all other organisms appear green (due to uptake of malachite green). Hence, mycobacteria are called acid-fast bacilli. A fluorescent stain, the auramine stain, can also be used to detect mycobacteria in specimens. It has the advantage that organisms can more easily be seen, as they fluoresce green against a black background. The medium is called Löwenstein–Jensen (L–J) medium. Most mycobacteria are slowly growing organisms compared to other bacteria and may take 2–12 weeks before producing visible growth on the medium. *Mycobacterium leprae* cannot be cultured on artificial media.

2 The clinical presentation of the patient is suggestive of tuberculosis, the most important mycobacterial cause of which is *M. tuberculosis*. The identity cannot be determined from an examination of the Ziehl–Neelsen stain, nor entirely from the characteristics of the growth on the L–J medium. Once growth is obtained, the organism's identity must be established by a series of microbiological and biochemical tests. Additionally, sensitivity tests are performed on the organism. Because of the organism's slow growth, it may be several months from taking the original specimen before the organism's identity and sensitivity can be established. Tuberculosis is therefore a clinical diagnosis and treatment should be started as soon as the diagnosis is made and not delayed for microbiological confirmation.

3 Detection of mycobacteria in clinical samples can be more rapidly achieved using an automated, radiometric culture technique, (BACTEC 460), when compared to culture on L–J medium. Specimens decontaminated in the same way as for culture on L–J medium are inoculated into a broth containing carbon-14(^{14}C) palmitic acid, which is metabolized by mycobacteria to yield $^{14}CO_2$. The evolution of $^{14}CO_2$ is detected in the BACTEC 460 instrument. Even more rapid detection of *M. tuberculosis* in clinical samples can be achieved with the polymerase chain reaction (PCR). The use of monoclonal antibodies specific to mycobacterial antigens in order to detect rapidly *M. tuberculosis* is giving encouraging results.

4 Standard triple therapy for pulmonary tuberculosis is a combination of rifampicin, isoniazid and pyrazinamide given for 2 months, followed

7   by a further 4 months of treatment with rifampicin and isoniazid. In some cases ethambutol can be added in the initial phase of treatment if resistance to isoniazid, is likely. Because of the length of treatment, non-compliance is a problem, which is in part leading to the development of multidrug-resistant *M. tuberculosis*, particularly in major cities in the USA and Africa.

    If the patient remains in hospital, she should be kept in isolation for the first 2 weeks of treatment. The consultant in communicable diseases control (CCDC) should be informed and the patient's contacts traced.

    Vaccination against infection with *M. tuberculosis* can be given using a live attenuated strain of *M. bovis* (bacillus Calmette-Guérin or BCG vaccination), which achieves over 70% protection and is given as part of a schedule of routine immunization in schools at the age of 10–14 years.

References

Mitchison DA (1992) Understanding the chemotherapy of tuberculosis – current problems. *J. Antimicrob. Chemother.* **29**, 477–493.

Uttley AHC & Pozniak A (1993) Resurgence of tuberculosis. *J. Hosp. Infect.* **23**, 249–253.

Young LS (1993) Mycobacterial diseases in the 1990s. *J. Antimicrob. Chemother.* **32**, 179–194.

A 20-year-old patient with cystic fibrosis was admitted to hospital with a 8 temperature and purulent sputum 1 week following a visit to a special holiday camp for patients with cystic fibrosis. A sputum was sent to the laboratory for microscopy (Fig. 8.1) and culture. The Gram-negative organism was identified as *Pseudomonas cepacia*.

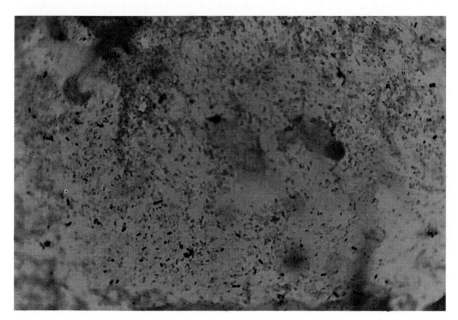

Fig. 8.1

Questions
1 What is the significance of this finding?
2 What other pulmonary infections do these patients get?
3 What other infections are assocated with *Pseudomonas*?

8 Answers

1 Colonization of the respiratory tract of patients with cystic fibrosis by *P. cepacia* can be asymtomatic in some, but may lead to severe deterioration of respiratory function (with a necrotizing pneumonia and septicaemia) in other patients. Females are more at risk of infection. The organism has a wide environmental reservoir, being found particularly in vegetation, where it is a recognized plant pathogen. Person-to-person transmission is the most likely route of infection, although infection from contaminated equipment may also occur. In order to diminish acquisition of the organism by non-colonized patients, segregation of patients at clinics, during physiotherapy and separate holiday camps for colonized and non-colonized patients has been advocated. *P. cepacia* is resistant to many antibiotics and thus treatment of infected patients is difficult and depends upon the sensitivity of the isolate.

2 Patients with cystic fibrosis also develop pulmonary infections with *Staphylococcus aureus* and mucoid strains of *P. aeruginosa*.

3 Pseudomonads are environmental organisms that are principal causes of nosocomial infection. *P. aeruginosa* is the most commonly isolated species. They are often associated with urinary tract infections in catheterized patients or respiratory infections in patients on ventilators. *P. aeruginosa* is also associated with an endophthalmitis, linked to the use of contaminated contact lenses, a destructive otitis externa and folliculitis, linked to the use of jacuzzis. In addition to *P. cepacia*, mucoid strains of *P. aeruginosa* also cause respiratory infections in patients with cystic fibrosis.

   P. pseudomallei is the cuase of melioidosis and *P. mallei* the cause of glanders. Melioidosis is a disseminated infection with widespread abscesses in the skin and organs of the body. It may also present in a similar fashion to tuberculosis. The infection is endemic in Asia and northern Australia and is contracted by the organism gaining entry to the body through skin abrasions from contaminated soil. Glanders presents in a similar fashion to melioidosis and is caught by contact with infected horses.

References

Editorial (1992) *Pseudomonas cepacia* – more than a harmless commensal. *Lancet* **339**, 1385–1386.

Goven JRW & Glass S (1990) The microbiology and therapy of cystic fibrosis lung infections. *Rev. Med. Microbiol.* **11**, 19–28.

A patient was neutropenic 1 week after a bone marrow transplantation, **9** when he developed a temperature. Blood cultures were taken before the patient was commenced on broad-spectrum antibiotics (an aminoglycoside and a β-lactam). An *Escherichia coli* was isolated from the blood culture. The patient's temperature responded shortly after starting the antibiotics but after a few days a low-grade temperature developed and diffuse opacities were noted on a chest X-ray. The patient was still on the antibiotics. A nose swab taken 1 week previously had grown the organism shown in Fig. 9.1.

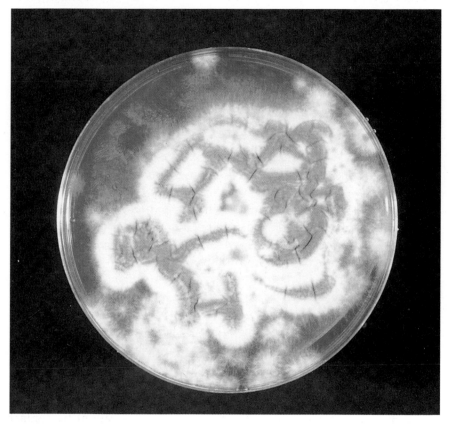

Fig. 9.1

Questions
1 What is the organism isolated from the nose swab and what relevance could it have to the patient's illness?
2 How should the patient be managed?

9 Answers

1 The organism is *Aspergillus fumigatus*. This is a mycelial fungus which is widespread in the environment. The organism is slow-growing and takes 3–4 days to produce visible growth on Sabouraud's medium. There are about 100 species of *Aspergillus* but, in addition to *A. fumigatus*, only a few have been implicated in causing human disease, for example, *A. flavus*, *A. niger* and *A. terreus*.

   A. fumigatus is associated with a number of distinct illnesses. Hypersensitivity to *A. fumigatus* causes allergic aspergillosis, which may present as asthma, and the patient may have eosinophils in the sputum and elevated immunoglobulin E (IgE) levels. *Aspergillus* may colonize a cavity in a lung, to produce an aspergilloma or fungal ball growing in the cavity. This may be asymptomatic or produce haemoptysis. Invasive aspergillosis can occur in immunocompromised patients, as in this case, where the fungus grows in the lung tissue, producing a sequestrum of dead tissue. These patients are prone to severe haemoptysis. *Aspergillus* may also cause infection of the paranasal sinuses and the outer ear, to produce destructive lesions in both areas. Ulcerative tracheobronchitis has recently been established as another clinical condition caused by *A. fumigatus* in patients with AIDS.

   Aspergillus spores are found in the air and immunocompromised individuals are easily colonized. Colonization can be detected by taking nose swabs. Large numbers of spores are found in proximity to building works, which can act as a source of infection for compromised patients.

2 Because severe haemoptysis can occur with invasive aspergillosis, surgery should be considered; otherwise, invasive aspergillosis is treated with amphotericin B. Amphotericin B is nephrotoxic and the side-effects of treatment may be diminished by giving the antifungal in a liposomal preparation. As an alternative, itraconazole is effective against *Aspergillus*.

References

Maartens G & Wood MJ (1991) The clinical presentation and diagnosis of invasive fungal infections. *J. Antimicrob. Chemother.* **28** (Suppl.), 13–22.

Working Party Report (1993) Chemoprophylaxis for candidosis and aspergillosis in neutropenia and transplantation: a review and recommendations. *J. Antimicrob. Chemother.* **32**, 5–21.

A 9-month-old child developed a respiratory illness with fever and a cough. Sputum was unavailable for culture and viral studies for respiratory syncytial virus were negative. A per-nasal swab taken for bacteriological culture grew the organism shown in Fig. 10.1. A Gram stain was prepared from the culture (Fig. 10.2). Subsequently, the patient developed paroxysmal coughing with inspiratory stridor, apnoeic attacks, cyanosis and vomiting. Conjuctival haemorrhages were caused by the paroxysmal coughing.

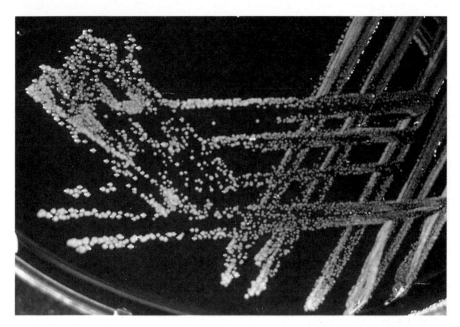

Fig. 10.1

10

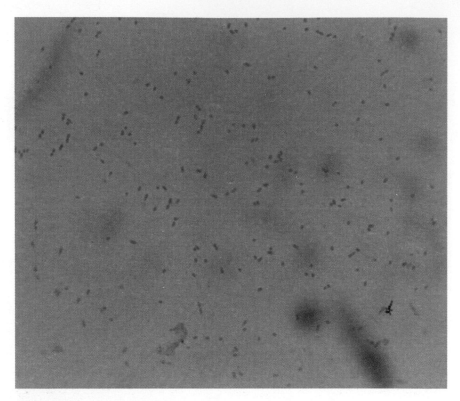

Fig. 10.2

Questions
1 What is the likely identity of the organism?
2 What special conditions are required for the culture of this organism?
3 Are antibiotics of any value in this condition?
4 What virulence properties does this organism have?

Answers

1 Clinically the patient has whooping cough, which is caused by *Bordetella pertussis*. The prodromal catarrhal phase is followed by the paroxysmal phase and, with progressive diminution in the frequency of paroxysms, the recovery phase. During the paroxysmal stage the child may develop bronchopneumonia, pneumothorax or even cerebral haemorrhage. The child is particularly infectious during the catarrhal phase, but infection lasts for about 3 weeks from the onset of illness. The organism colonizes respiratory epithelium and is transmitted by droplet infection.

2 The organism is very difficult to recover from patients when the paroxysmal and clinically distinctive stage has started. Diagnosis is often serological and therefore retrospective. Per-nasal swabs have a high sensitivity for detecting *B. pertussis*, but cough plates, where a plate of culture medium is held in front of the child as it coughs or sneezes, can also be used. Culture requires a medium that contains penicillin, to inhibit normal oropharyngeal flora, and charcoal to neutralize toxic substances that may inhibit growth of the organism.

3 If given early enough in the course of the illness, erythromycin may reduce the severity of the disease. The disease can be prevented by vaccination with a killed suspension of *B. pertussis*. The vaccine is usually given as a triple vaccine combined with diphtheria and tetanus at 2, 3 and 4 months of age.

4 *B. pertussis* produces a number of potential virulence factors. Pertussis toxin (PT), produced only by *B. pertussis*, has adenosine triphosphate (ATP)-ribosyltransferase activity, whose target is the guanosine triphosphate (GTP)-binding protein of the membrane adenylate-cyclase complex of mammalian cells. Together with the filamentous haemagglutinin (FHA), it mediates the binding of *B. pertussis* to respiratory epithelial cells. Both PT and FHA are components of the modern acellular vaccine. *Bordetella* also produces adenylate cyclate toxin, which has a number of inhibitory effects upon immune cells. It elevates intracellular cyclic adenosine monophosphate (cAMP) levels. Tracheal cytotoxin is produced by all species of *Bordetella* and has a selective destructive effect upon ciliated cells, inhibiting DNA synthesis. Heat-labile toxin induces vasoconstriction and is dermonecrotic in action. The cell wall of *Bordetella* is composed in part of lipopolysaccharide

10   (endotoxin), which has the same pathophysiological effects as other Gram-negative bacteria.

Reference

Nelson JD (1978) The changing epidemiology of pertussis in young infants—the role of adults as reservoirs of infection. *Am. J. Dis. Child.* **32**, 371–374.

A 20-year-old man had been complaining of sudden onset of headache, neck stiffness and that the light hurt his eyes (photophobia). He was admitted to hospital, and found to have a haemorrhagic skin rash, neck rigidity and a positive Kernig's sign. He did not have papilloedema. His white blood count was 30 × 10^9/l with a normal differential count. A lumbar puncture was performed, the cerebrospinal fluid (CSF) centrifuged and a Gram stain was performed on the deposit (Fig. 11.1).

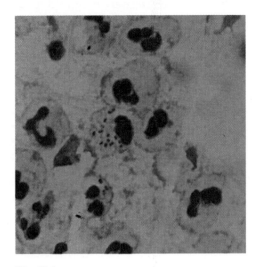

Fig. 11.1

Questions
1 What is the most likely identity of the organism?
2 What do you expect the white count in the CSF to be?
3 With which antibiotic should the patient be treated?
4 What public health measures should be taken?

Answers

1 Clinically the patient has meninigitis. Meningitis is caused by viruses (aseptic), bacteria or fungi. The microbiological cause of meningitis is determined by measuring the biochemical and cellular changes in the CSF and detecting the presence of the causative organism. The bacterial causes of meningitis generally correlate with the age of the patient. Neonatal meningitis is usually caused by *Escherichia coli* and Lancefield group B streptococcus; meningitis in childhood is caused by *Streptococcus pneumoniae*, *Neisseria meningitidis* and *Haemophilus influenzae*; meningitis in adults by *N. meningitidis*; and meningitis in the elderly by *S. pneumoniae*. Other bacterial causes of meningitis are *Listeri a monocytogenes*, often in immunocompromised individuals, *Staphylococcus aureus* associated with head injury, *Leptospira* and *Mycobacterium tuberculosis*. In this case, Fig. 11.1 shows numerous Gram-negative cocci in pairs, located within the cytoplasm of the pus cells. The organism is therefore likely to be *N. meningitidis*. *N. meningitidis* can be subdivided into serogroups A, B, C, W135, 29E, X, Y and Z, based upon the capsular polysaccharide. Serogroups B and C can be further subdivided into serotypes based upon the antigenicity of outer-membrane proteins. The commonest serogroups causing disease in the UK are B (two-thirds) and C (one-third), with very small numbers of cases caused by Y, W135 and A. Currently, the commonest type is B15 P1:16. *N. meningitidis* can also cause a chronic septicaemia and pyogenic arthritis. The other important pathogen belonging to this genus is *N. gonorrhoeae*.

2 This is a case of pyogenic (bacterial) meningitis. The CSF is usually purulent, with a white blood cell (WBC) count varying from 100 to over 1000 cells/mm^3 with a predominance of polymorphonuclear leucocytes (PMN); the CSF glucose concentration will be slightly reduced, below 3.0 mmol/l, and generally will be less than 50% of a simultaneous serum glucose estimation; the CSF protein levels will be elevated (0.5–1.0 g/l).

In aseptic, leptospiral and cryptococcal meningitis there will be an elevated WBC count (10–500/mm^3) with a predominance of lymphocytes, the CSF glucose concentration will be normal but the protein concentration will be slightly increased (0.5–1.0 g/l).

In tuberculous meningitis the cellular response will be similar to aseptic meningitis but the glucose level will be very much reduced and may be undetectable. The protein level will be increased (1.0–6.0 g/l).

In this case a Gram stain has revealed the presence of *N. meningitidis*.

If tuberculous meningitis is suspected, a Ziehl–Neelsen stain would be performed; if cryptococcal meningitis, an Indian ink (negative stain) preparation made; and if leptospiral meningitis, the organism may be detected by dark ground microscopy. As well as microscopy, the CSF specimen is cultured on chocolate agar (or if tuberculosis is suspected, on Löwenstein–Jensen medium) and any organism that grows is identified and sensitivity tests performed.

For *S. pneumoniae*, *N. meningitidis*, *H. influenzae* and *Cryptococcus neoformans*, latex agglutination tests exist for the rapid detection of the organism in the CSF. Apart from their speed, these tests are useful when prior antibiotics have been given and culture may be unhelpful.

3 Benzylpenicillin. This antibiotic is likely to be active against the two most common causes of bacterial meningitis, *N. meningitidis* and *S. pneumoniae*. The speed with which treatment is instituted often determines the success of treatment and one dose of benzylpenicillin should be carried by every general practitioner so that treatment can be started as soon as bacterial meningitis is suspected, even though this may prejudice the growth of the organism from the CSF. An alternative empiric therapy for meningitis is chloramphenicol, and this is preferable if the patient is between 1 and 5 years as *H. influenzae* is common in this age group.

The first choices of antibiotic for other bacterial causes of meningitis are *E. coli* (cefotaxime), Lancefield group B streptococcus (benzylpenicillin), *Leptospira* (benzylpenicillin), *H. influenzae* (amoxycillin, ceftriaxone or, if a β-lactamase producer, chloramphenicol), *Listeria* (amoxycillin), *S. aureus* (flucloxacillin), *M. tuberculosis* (triple therapy).

A vaccine exists which protects against illness caused by groups A and C, but not B. This vaccine should be given to travellers to endemic areas.

Immunization against *H. influenzae* type b (Hib) disease is currently part of the childhood immunization schedule.

A vaccine against severe *S. pneumoniae* disease also exists, but there is no evidence that secondary illness following contact with an index case of *S. pneumoniae* meninigitis occurs and the vaccine is not indicated for this purpose.

11 **4** *N. meningitidis* is notifiable and the case should be reported to the consultant in communicable disease control.

The patient should be admitted to hospital and the source isolated.

Close contacts should have chemoprophylaxis with rifampicin or ciprofloxacin. The use of nasopharyngeal swabs to detect carriage is controversial.

If the patient has meningitis caused by *H. influenzae*, close household childhood contacts have a greatly increased risk of developing secondary disease.

References
Editorial (1990) Preventing meningococcal infection. *Drug Ther. Bull.* **28**, 34–36.

Lambert HP (1989) Unresolved problems in meningitis. *J. Antimicrob. Chemother.* **24**, 978–1002.

A woman had spontaneous rupture of membranes at 32/40 weeks' ges- **12** tation. After 24 h the neonate became pyrexial and distressed. A blood specimen was taken for culture (Fig. 12.1) which after 24 hours was positive and a Gram stain was performed. The same organism was isolated from the cerebrospinal fluid (CSF).

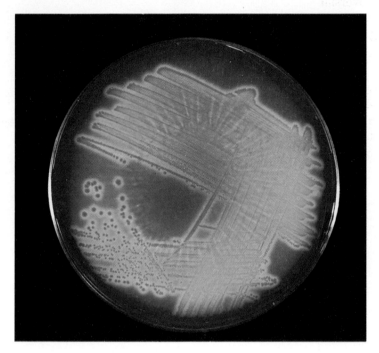

Fig. 12.1

12

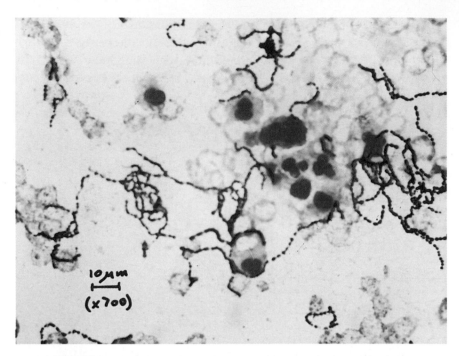

Fig. 12.2

Questions

1 What is the likely identity of the organism and what other organisms typically cause meningitis in this age group?
2 How may this organism by typed and what is the clinical significance of the type?
3 What factors predispose to meningitis with this organism?
4 How should the patient be treated?

1 The most likely identity of the organism is *Streptococcus agalactiae* (β-haemolytic streptococcus, Lancefield group B). The Gram stain of the blood culture demonstrates that it is a Gram-positive coccus and the organism is β-haemolytic on blood agar. Group B streptococcus is the commonest cause of meningitis in this age group. Meningitis caused by group B streptococcus usually presents within the first few days of life as a general systemic infection with respiratory distress and without obvious signs of meningitis. Meningeal involvement occurs in about 30% of neonatal disease caused by *S. agalactiae* within the first day or two of life. *S. agalactiae* also causes meningitis in neonates who are a few days older. Although disease occurring within a day or two of birth is predominantly septicaemic, the presentation of group B-associated disease at about 10 days of age is more typically a clinical presentation of meningitis.

2 Seven capsular serotypes of group B streptococcus exist—Ia, Ib, II, III, IV, V and VI—based upon cell-wall carbohydrate. The septicaemic illness occurring within a day or two of birth reflects the prevalence of the capsular types and is caused principally by types Ia, Ib and II. Type III is responsible for over 80% of all cases of meningitis, whether occurring as part of the septicaemic illness within a day or two of birth, or a few days later. Early-onset disease is acquired from the mother during birth; late-onset disease is acquired from environmental sources within the nursery or cross-contamination from other infected neonates.

3 Early-onset disease can only occur if there is maternal carriage of the organism at birth. The prevalence of maternal carriage varies widely but is of the order of 25% and can vary through the duration of pregnancy.

   The risk of early-onset disease is related to the heaviness of maternal colonization and the risk is increased if there is prolonged rupture of membrane, amnionitis or prematurity of the neonate. As a risk factor, prematurity may be related to physiological low levels of complement factors. Lack of maternal antibodies against type III capsular polysaccharide is also a risk factor.

4 Treatment should be with penicillin and gentamicin.

   There are two approaches to prevention of neonatal early-onset group B disease. The first is prophylaxis and the second is vaccination.

12 In areas of high prevalence of neonatal disease caused by *S. agalactiae* (e.g. the USA), a mass screening policy is adopted, with prophylaxis during labour, using ampicillin, in those mothers who have identifiable risk factors. In areas of low prevalence of disease (e.g. the UK), an alternative approach is to identify mothers who have risk factors and use rapid detection methods to determine carriage of group B streptococcus and then give prophylaxis.

Currently, capsular type III carbohydrate–protein conjugates are being developed and tested as potential vaccines.

References

Van Oppen C & Feldman R (1993) Antibiotic prophylaxis of neonatal group B streptococcal infections. *Br. Med. J.* **306**, 411–412.

Wessels MR & Kasper DL (1993) The changing spectrum of group B streptococcal disease. *N. Engl. J. Med.* **328**, 1843–1844.

A 4-year-old child became unwell over a period of a few days with a temperature, headache and photophobia. The child was admitted to hospital where a blood culture and cerebrospinal fluid (CSF) specimen (Fig. 13.1) were taken. The child did not have a rash.

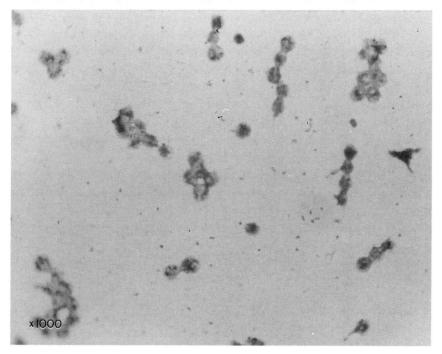

Fig. 13.1

Questions
1 What is the likely identity of the organism and how may it be confirmed?
2 What other illnesses are caused by members of this genus? What other illnesses does this organism cause in this age group?
3 How should the patient be managed? What public health consequences are there of this child becoming infected?
4 How may this illness be prevented?

13 Answers

1 Meningitis occurring in a 4-year-old child with small Gram-negative rods in the CSF is most likely to be due to *Haemophilus influenzae*. This can be confirmed by isolation of the organism from the CSF on 'chocolate' agar (blood agar heated in order to lyse the erythrocytes and release growth factors that are required by *Haemophilus* species). The identity of the organism can be established by demonstrating its cultural requirements for both haemin (X factor) and nicotinamide adenine dinucleotide (NAD; V factor). The presence of the organism may also be detected in the CSF by rapid antigen detection methods using antibody-coated latex particles. Similar rapid antigen detection methods are used for meningitis caused by *Streptococcus pneumoniae*, *Neisseria meningitidis*, *Escherichia coli* and *Cryptococcus neoformans*. Soluble capsular antigen can also be detected in serum or urine in cases of meningitis.

　　H. influenzae may be either capsulate or non-capsulate. Most invasive disease is caused by capsulate organisms. There are six capsular types—Pitman types a–f. Pitman type b is the most common type causing disease. Apart from meningitis, other severe invasive diseases may occur with *H. influenzae*, such as orbital cellulitis, epiglottitis, pyogenic arthritis and osteomyelitis. Non-capsulate *H. influenzae* are a cause of sinusitis, otitis media or exacerbation of chronic bronchitis, along with *S. pneumoniae*, and can occur at any age.

2 Species of *Haemophilus* other than *H. influenzae* are also the cause of disease. *H. ducreyi* (X factor-dependent) is the cause of chancroid. This is a sexually transmitted disease that is prevalent in tropical countries. It presents with indurated ulcers on the genitals with associated regional lymphadenopathy which may ulcerate. The organism can be isolated from scrapings of the ulcer and the disease is treated with tetracycline.

　　Endocarditis can be caused by *H. influenzae*, *H. aphrophilis* and *H. parainfluenzae*, although they are rare.

3 The patient should be treated with ampicillin. In areas where the prevalence of ampicillin resistance is high, then chloramphenicol, cefotaxime or ceftriaxone may be used. However, the prevalence of chloramphenicol resistance in *H. influenzae* is also increasing. In a recent survey of ampicillin resistance in the UK, only 7% of isolates were resistant, although in some countries, for example, Spain, the prevalence may be as high as 50% (Campos *et al.* 1984).

H. influenzae type b disease occurs at an increased frequency in households where there is a primary case. This frequency is age-related and is greatest in children under 2 years of age. The route of transmission is either by droplet infection or contact with nasopharyngeal secretions and the source of infection is either the infected primary case or an asymptomatic carrier, for example, the mother. Ampicillin or chloramphenicol does not eradicate nasopharyngeal carriage and the close contacts of this case should be given chemoprophylaxis. It is arguable that all household contacts, irrespective of age, should be given rifampicin 20 mg/kg to a maximum of 600 mg daily or the appropriate paediatric dose for 4 days. The evidence for an increased risk of secondary disease to playgroup and schoolroom contacts of index cases is poor and prophylaxis is not recommended unless more than one case occurs within the group.

4 Invasive *H. influenzae* group b disease can be prevented by vaccination. Several different vaccines exist which are conjugates of polyribosyl-ribitol phosphate and carrier proteins. The commercially available vaccines differ in the carrier protein used as adjuvant, whether diphtheria toxoid, non-toxigenic mutant of diphtheria toxin, tetanus toxoid or the outer membrane protein of *N. meningitidis* group B. Once a course of vaccination is started with one vaccine it should be continued with the same vaccine. *H. influenzae* type b (Hib) vaccine should be given along with the primary diphtheria/tetanus/pertussis course at 2, 3 and 4 months of age.

References

Campos J *et al.* (1984) Antimicrobial Agents. *Chemotherapy* **23**, 706–709.
Shapiro ED (1990) New vaccines against *H. influenzae* type b. *Pediatr. Clin. North Am.* **37**, 567–583.
Turk DC (1984) The pathogenicity of *H. influenzae*. *J. Med. Microbiol.* **18**, 1–18.

14 A patient who was receiving immunosuppressive therapy following a renal transplantation became pyrexial, complained of a headache and had an epileptic attack. As the patient did not have papilloedema, a cerebrospinal fluid (CSF) specimen was taken for culture and microscopy. The white cell count was 1000/mm³ (79% polymorphs), the protein was 1.0 g/l and the glucose 3.0 mmol/l. Organisms were not seen on the Gram stain. An organism was isolated from the CSF, a subculture of which is shown in Fig. 14.1 and a Gram stain of the culture is shown in Fig. 14.2. The same organism was isolated from the blood culture.

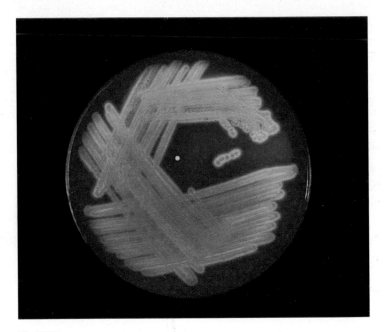

Fig. 14.1

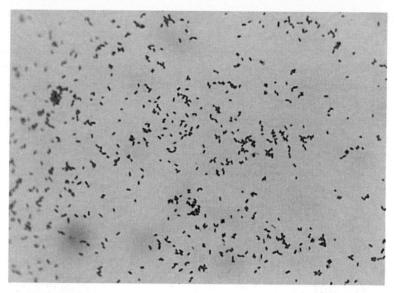

Fig. 14.2

Questions

1 What is your diagnosis?
2 What is the source of infection for this organism?
3 How should the patient be treated?
4 What other groups of people are susceptible to infection with this organism and how may infection be prevented?

Answers

1 This immunocompromised patient has meningitis caused by *Listeria monocytogenes*. Organisms are few in the CSF and the Gram stain may be negative in 60% of cases. The typical cellular response is of a pyogenic meningitis with elevated protein and white cell response, mainly polymorphs. In *Listeria* infection of the meninges, the glucose levels are normal in more than 60% of cases, unlike other bacterial infections. *Listeria* infections in the central nervous system (CNS) often present with signs of a meningoencephalitis or abscess formation, and the patient may have ataxia or fits. The blood culture is also positive in 60% of cases.

   L. monocytogenes is a Gram-positive rod (Fig. 14.2) and β-haemolytic on blood agar (Fig. 14.1). It grows over a wide temperature range and can grow slowly at 4°C. There are seven species of *Listeria* but *L. monocytogenes* is the only human pathogen. It is an intracellular pathogen and immunity is mainly T-cell-mediated. Intracellularly the organism precipitates actin filaments and causes cytoskeletal changes. It may be confused with diphtheroids and be ignored as a contaminant. If a suspension of a culture is looked at microscopically, the organisms have a characteristic end-over-end tumbling motility.

2 *L. monocytogenes* has a wide environmental reservoir and is found in water and soil and on vegetation. It is also found widely in many species of animal, for example, sheep, cattle, birds and fish, and high counts of the organism have been detected in a variety of soft cheeses and sausage meat. The source of human infection is contaminated foods, mainly dairy products.

3 *L. monocytogenes* is sensitive to a wide range of antibiotics. A combination of ampicillin and gentamicin is considered to be the treatment of choice. In patients who are hypersensitive to β-lactams, co-trimoxazole can be used.

4 *Listeria* infection is most commonly associated with the third trimester of pregnancy. The infection may present as a flu-like illness. Transplacental infection of the fetus can lead to abortion or birth of an infected infant, which is characterized by widespread granuloma, for example, in spleen, skin and liver. The organism can also be isolated from granuloma in the placenta. Early-onset listeriosis can be prevented by modifying the woman's diet during pregnancy, omitting food

known to be heavily contaminated with *Listeria*, for example, soft cheeses. Late-onset listeriosis in infancy occurs several weeks after birth and presents as meningitis.

Up to 30% of sporadic cases of non-pregnancy-associated *Listeria* infection can occur in adults who have no obvious predisposing causes, such as immunosuppression, as in this case. The presentation in these cases is mainly with meningitis. Epidemics of *Listeria* infection have been reported, linked to consumption of infected dairy products or coleslaw, where both pregnant females and non-pregnant adults were affected.

References
Gellin BG & Broome CV (1989) Listeriosis. *J. A. M. A.* **261**, 1313–1320.
Schuchat A, Swaminathan B & Broome CV (1991) Epidemiology of human listeriosis. *Clin. Microbiol. Rev.* **4**, 169–183.

15 A man was found comatose and admitted to hospital. Relatives reported that he suffered from chronic otitis media and that they had noticed increasing confusion over some days before his admission. A computerised tomography (CT) scan of his skull was performed; it showed a lesion consistent with an abscess in the temporal lobe. Material aspirated from the abscess was Gram-stained (Fig. 15.1) and cultured.

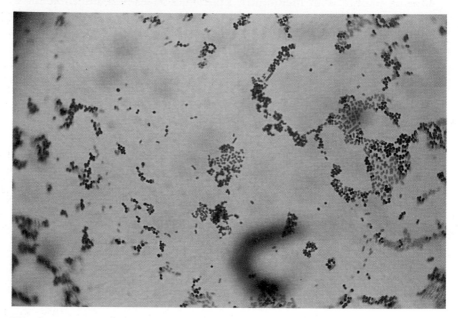

Fig. 15.1

Questions
1 Are the microbiological findings unusual?
2 What rapid tests exist that can influence therapy?
3 What is the management?

1 No. The most likely source of infection in this case is the chronic middle-ear infection, which is a common predisposing factor for brain abscesses. Abscesses of otic origin are most often found in the adjacent temporal lobe and are frequently mixed, as in this case. The microbiology of otogenic brain abscess is often a mixture of aerobic and anaerobic organism—frequently streptococci and most frequently *Streptococcus milleri* (the Gram-positive coccus in Fig. 15.1) or Gramnegative aerobic bacteria, for example, *Proteus* with anaerobic organism—*Bacteroides* or *Fusobacterium*, most commonly (the Gramnegative bacillus in Fig. 15.1). Abscesses secondary to dental or sinus infections are also frequently mixed (streptococci and Gram-negative anaerobes). Abscesses secondary to trauma are often caused by *Staphylococcus aureus*.

    S. milleri is a viridans streptococcus that is part of the normal oropharyngeal flora. It belongs to Lancefield group F (Lancefield grouping is not restricted to β-haemolytic streptococci) and is often a cause of abscess in many organs, for example, liver, lung, brain, etc. *Bacteroides* and *Fusobacterium* are non-sporing anaerobic Gram-negative organisms that are part of the normal flora of the gastrointestinal tract and oropharynx. They also commonly cause abscesses, chronic sinusitis and otitis media.

2 Anaerobic bacteria derive their metabolic energy by fermentation and the volatile short-chain, fatty acid end-products of fermentation, for example, propionic and butyric acid, can be detected in pus and used to indicate the presence of anaerobic organisms. The volatile acids are detected by gas–liquid chromatography (GLC) and can be detected within an hour, whereas culture of anaerobic organisms takes 48 h. It is an important practical point that if pus is drained from any abscess it should *not* be discarded down the sluice in preference for a swab dipped in the pus to be sent to the microbiology department. The correct specimen to send for microbiological analysis is the pus.

3 If anaerobes are suspected in an abscess or if their presence is demonstrated by GLC of the pus, metronidazole should be given. For polymicrobial infections, penicillin should be added if streptococci are present (as in this case) or cefatoxime if aerobic Gram-negative bacteria are suspected. An alternative broad-spectrum antibiotic is chloramphenicol, although the concentration in pus can be erratic. The

15   treatment can be amended once the organisms have been grown and their sensitivity determined. Appropriate antibiotic treatment should be combined with surgical treatment, which is either drainage or excision through a craniotomy.

References

DeLouvois J, Gortval P & Hurley R (1977) Bacteriology of abscesses of the central nervous system: a multi centre prospective study. *Br. Med. J.* **2**, 981–984.

Seydoux C & Francioli P (1992) Bacterial brain absesses: factors influencing mortality and sequelae. *Clin. Infect. Dis.* **15**, 394–401.

A patient with AIDS was admitted to hospital giving a 1-week history of an intermittent temperature, headache, fits and an altered personality. A computerised tomography (CT) scan of his head was performed; this showed some cerebral atrophy but no focal lesions. A cerebrospinal fluid (CSF) specimen was taken for microscopy (Fig. 16.1) and culture.

16

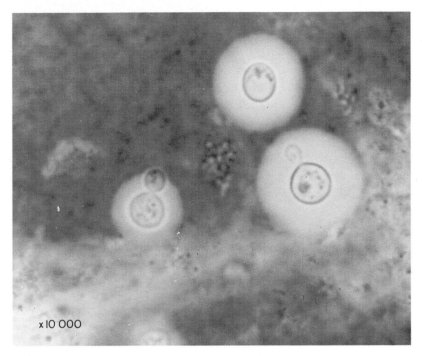

Fig. 16.1 Reprinted with the permission of Times
Mirror International publications

Questions

1 What is your diagnosis?
2 How may this infection also be diagnosed?
3 What is the likely source for this organism?
4 How should the patient be treated?

16 Answers

1 Figure 16.1 is an Indian ink preparation of the CSF and shows capsulate, budding yeasts. The ink acts as a negative stain, providing a dark background against which the yeast can be seen, surrounded by a thick capsule. The most likely identity of the yeast is *Cryptococcus neoformans*. This is the most frequent fungal cause of meningitis in patients with AIDS. The large capsule is also characteristic of *C. neoformans*. Its identity is established by culture and biochemical testing of the isolate.

   Cryptococcal meningitis is usually of slow onset, similar to meningitis caused by *Mycobacterium tuberculosis*. The organism can infect sites other than the meninges. Focal lesions can develop in the brain (cryptococcomas), lungs or skin.

2 The CSF usually shows a decreased glucose and elevated protein concentration with a predominant lymphocytic cellular response. Diagnosis can also be made by a latex agglutination test of either the CSF or serum.

3 The organism has an environmental reservoir and is found worldwide in soil. It is also found in pigeon faeces. Except very rarely, person-to-person transmission has not been reported. Recurrence of infection is due to relapse rather than reinfection.

4 Amphotericin and 5-flucytosine (5FC) is regarded by many as the treatment of choice, although the antifungal azoles, fluconazole and itraconazole, have been used with success. Amphotericin and 5FC is associated with a failure rate of 20–30% and in these circumstances fluconazole may be successful. Comparative trials of amphotericin versus azoles show equivalent response rates for both treatments. Some clinical factors at presentation suggest a poor prognosis – coma – a high titre of cryptococcal antigen and low numbers of white cells in the CSF. Azoles are cheaper and have fewer side-effects compared to amphotericin. For maintenance therapy after an attack of cryptococcal meningitis, the azoles are to be preferred because of ease of administration and lack of side-effects.

References

16

Buxtan MJ, Dubois DJ, Turner RR, Sculpher MJ, Robinson DA & Searcy C (1991) Cost implications of alternative treatments for AIDS patients with cryptococcal meningitis. Comparison of fluconazole and amphotericin based therapies. *J. Hosp. Infect.* **23**, 17–31.

Clark RA, Green D, Alkinson W, Valainis GT & Hyslop N (1990) Spectrum of *Cryptococcus neoformans* infection in 68 patients infected with HIV. *Rev. Infect. Dis.* **12**, 768–777.

17 A group of cadets developed cellulitis on their backs and arms 24 h after exercise in a gymnasium. Skin swabs were taken from the abraded lesions for microscopy (Fig. 17.1) and culture (Fig. 17.2).

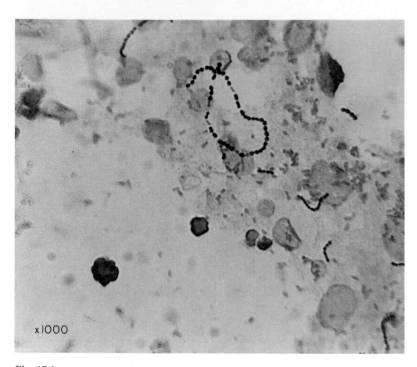

x 1000

Fig. 17.1

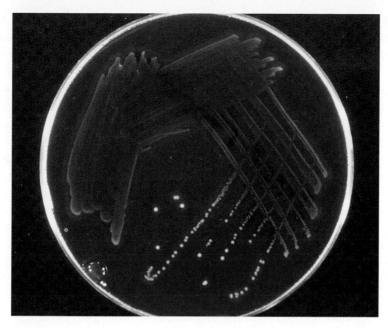

Fig. 17.2

Questions

1 How may this organism be typed and with what acute illnesses is it associated?
2 What serological markers can be useful for infections with this organism?
3 How was this organism transmitted in this instance?
4 What long-term sequelae may follow an infection with this organism?
5 How should the patients be treated?

17 Answers

1 This is a β-haemolytic streptococcus. Beta-haemolytic streptococci are divided into Lancefield groups based upon cell-wall carbohydrate antigens. Group A streptococci are called *Streptococcus pyogenes*, and they cause skin and throat infections and septicaemia; group B streptococci (*S. agalactiae*) are principally pathogens of neonates, causing meningitis and septicaemia; group C streptococci are animal-derived organisms that can cause sore throats and cellulitis; and group G streptococci cause similar clinical disease. Lancefield antigens are also found in (viridans) streptococci–*S. milleri* (group F) and in *Enterococcus* (previously *Streptococcus*) *faecalis* (group D). Other Lancefield antigens occur in streptococci of minor clinical importance.

   S. pyogenes (group A) can be subdivided into Griffiths types based upon cell-wall proteins. There are three cell-wall proteins produced by *S. pyogenes*–M, T and R. The M antigen is the most important and is a virulence factor with antiphagocytic properties.

   S. pyogenes produces a wide variety of extracellular products– streptolysin O and S, hyaluronidase, DNase, streptokinase and erythrogenic toxin.

   In addition to local infections of the skin and throat, *S. pyogenes* can cause puerperal sepsis, necrotizing fasciitis and septicaemia. It may also induce a number of acute toxin-induced illnesses. Scarlet fever may follow an infection with a strain of *S. pyogenes*, producing erythrogenic toxin. After a prodromal illness of a day or two the patient develops a characteristic erythematous rash on the torso and face but sparing the region around the mouth, thus producing a relative circumoral pallor. The tongue papillae become red and prominent, giving the typical 'strawberry' tongue. After a week, the skin begins to desquamate. The genetic locus coding for the erythrogenic toxin is *spe* A and is a virulence marker for serious invasive local or systemic disease carried by *S. pyogenes*, whether or not the patient develops clinical scarlet fever. The erythrogenic toxin is a superantigen, activating T cells in a non-antigen-dependent manner. Patients may also develop a toxic shock-like syndrome similar to that caused by enterotoxin B-producing *Staphylococcus aureus*.

2 Serological evidence of *S. pyogenes* infection can be obtained by determining the antistreptolysin O (ASO) and anti-DNase B titre of antibodies. In some infections of the skin the ASO titre may be within the normal range but the anti-DNase B titre is elevated.

3 *S. pyogenes* is transmitted by droplet infection or by direct contact. In this case the vehicle of transmission may have been the gymnasium equipment.

4 Three important long-term effects may follow an infection with *S. pyogenes*.

(a) Rheumatic fever—this is rarely seen today. It is probably caused by antibodies against the cell wall of the streptococcus and cross-reaction with connective tissue of the heart causing tissue destruction and distortion of the heart valve. The diagnosis of rheumatic fever is mainly clinical.

(b) Glomerulonephritis occurs 1–2 weeks following a *S. pyogenes* infection. This complication only follows with infections by certain nephritogenic M types, for example, M12, M25 in throat infections and M49 in skin infections. There is immunocomplex deposition in the basement membrane of the glomeruli, which leads to nephritis. The serum complement (C3) levels are decreased.

(c) Chorea—this is uncommon today.

5 The patient should be given benzylpenicillin. In hospital cases, patients should be source-isolated until the *S. pyogenes* has been eradicated.

References

Fischetti VA, Jones KF, Hollingshead SK & Scott JR (1988) Structure, function and genetics of streptococcal in protein. *Rev. Infect. Dis.* **10** (Suppl. 2), S356–S358.

Peter G & Smith A (1977) Group A streptococcal infections of the skin and pharynx. *N. Engl. J. Med.* **7**, 311–316 (part I), 365–370 (part II).

18 A diabetic was admitted to hospital with a pain in her foot. On examination, the foot was cold and pulses were absent. An emergency operation was performed which ended in a below-the-knee amputation. At 24 h after the operation the patient became hypotensive with a high temperature, red urine and pain at the operation site, which was noted to be distended and discharging a serosanguineous fluid, and crepitus was present. A swab was taken for microscopy (Fig. 18.1) and culture. The organism was subsequently plated across a lecithin–agar plate, one-half of which had been covered with antitoxin (Fig. 18.2).

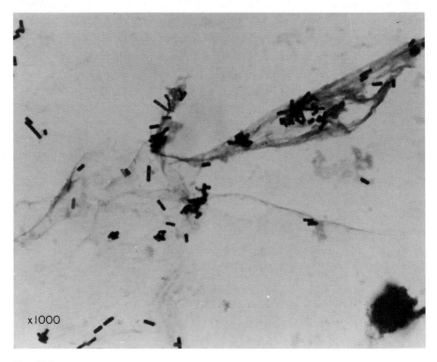

Fig. 18.1

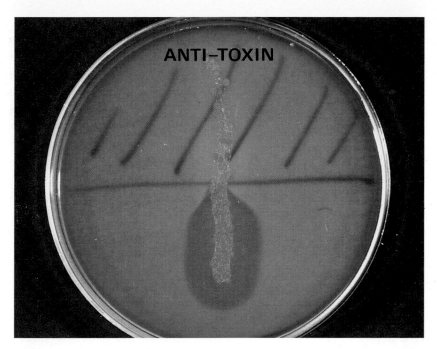

Fig. 18.2

Questions
1 What is your diagnosis?
2 How may this illness have been prevented?
3 How should the patient be managed?
4 Why is the patient's urine red?
5 What other illnesses do bacteria belonging to this genus cause?

18 Answers

1 The patient has gas gangrene. The typical features are the high temperature, shock and severe pain with local signs of oedema, gas formation, myonecrosis and discoloured skin overlying the infection. Gas gangrene is caused by clostridia, mainly *Clostridium perfringens*, although other clostridial species also cause gas gangrene. Clostridia are spore-producing anaerobic Gram-positive bacilli (Fig. 18.1) and are found in the faeces, from where they may contaminate the skin of the thighs. Clostridial spores inoculated into devitalized tissue with a poor blood supply may germinate. The bacteria multiply locally, producing many extraceullular products, which cause the toxic effects of gas gangrene. In this case the patient's blood supply to the leg had been occluded due to diabetic-induced arteriopathy. Gas gangrene may also follow traumatic injuries, both civilian and military.

2 Gas gangrene can be prevented by giving prophylactic benzylpenicillin before lower-limb amputation and following traumatic injury.

3 The most essential component of treatment is surgical debridement of all devitalized tissue. The patient should also be given benzylpenicillin and, depending upon the results of culture, antibiotics appropriate for any other bacteria that may be present. Hyperbaric oxygen can improve oxygenation of the tissue and help limit the gangrene. Antitoxin is generally not given because of the development of hypersensitivity reactions.

4 *C. perfringens* produces five major toxins and several minor toxins which have dermonecrotic and lethal effects. One of the toxins, called α-toxin, is a phospholipase C. Phospholipid is an important structural component of cell walls, particularly erythrocytes, and the phospholipase secreted into the patient's circulation causes haemolysis which can present as haemoglobinuria and discolour the urine red. The effect of α-toxin on lecithin is shown in Fig. 18.2, where the lecithin (from egg yolk) is hydrolysed and triglycerides are precipitated to produce an opalescent zone around the growth. This effect is inhibited by *C. perfringens* anti-α-toxin. This laboratory reaction is called the Nagler reaction.

5 The genus *Clostridium* comprises numerous species, several of which are important human pathogens.

In addition to causing gas gangrene, *C. perfringens* causes food poisoning. The illness has a 12–24-h incubation period and presents with colicky abdominal pain and diarrhoea. It is caused by eating inadequately cooked food, usually meat stews contaminated with large numbers of *C. perfringens*, that release enterotoxins into the gastrointestinal tract. The organism can be recovered in large numbers from the faeces or from the food. The toxin can be detected in the faeces by enzyme-linked immunosorbent assay (ELISA).

C. tetani causes tetanus. This illness usually follows contamination of a wound by the spores of the organism. The neurotoxin of *C. tetani* is a zinc endopeptidase. The site of action of the toxin is the inhibitory synapses in the spinal cord which modulate the motor reflex arc. The toxin reaches the spinal cord by axonal spread along the peripheral nerves and is taken up by the inhibitory nerves. The enzyme cleaves certain 'docking' proteins present on the vesicles containing the inhibitory neurotransmitter. The removal of the proteins from the surface of the vesicle prevents its fusion with the synaptic membrane, the release of the neurotransmitter and allows unrestricted stimulation of the reflex arc leading to muscle spasm.

Tetanus can be prevented by vaccination with a toxoid and is part of the childhood schedule given at 2, 3 and 4 months of age. In non-immunized patients who have an injury, wound debridement, prophylaxis with hyperimmune globulin and a first dose of a course of toxoid and penicillin should all be given.

C. botulinum causes botulism. This is a type of food poisoning and outbreaks have occurred following consumption of tins of salmon or hazelnut yoghurt that have been contaminated with the organism. The incubation period is 12–72h and the patient presents with diplopia, dysphonia, dysphagia and even respiratory paralysis. The illness is caused by the release of a neurotoxin that is a zinc endopeptidase. The enzyme acts in a similar fashion to tetanus toxin but prevents the fusion of the acetylcholine-containing synaptic vesicles with the synaptic membrane at the motor end-plate. The patient has a flaccid paralysis, unlike tetanus, where the patient has a spastic paralysis. There is no routine vaccination against botulism but antitoxin is used in treatment.

C. difficile causes pseudomembranous colitis which presents with abdominal pain, distention and bloody diarrhoea. Characteristic plaques can be seen in the colon at sigmoidoscopy. The illness is caused by two toxins and is treated with oral vancomycin or metronidazole.

18 Reference

Darke SG, King AM & Slack WK (1977) Gas gangrene and related infections: classification, clinical features and aetiology, management and mortality: a report of 88 cases. *Br. J. Surg.* **64**, 104–112.

Forty-eight hours postoperatively, two patients on one ward and another patient on a second ward all became pyrexial with signs of a local wound infection. Swabs were taken from the patients' wounds for microscopy (Fig. 19.1). The organism was identified as *Staphylococcus aureus* and phage-typed (Fig. 19.2).

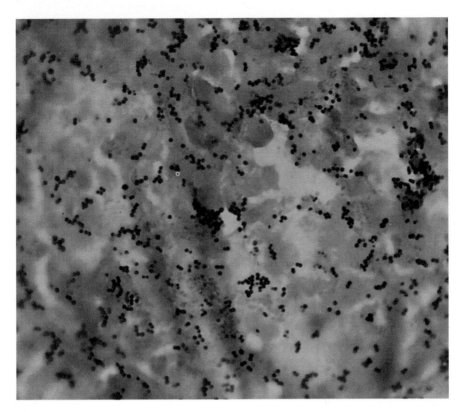

Fig. 19.1

Source of isolate	29	52	52a	79	80	3a	3c	55	71	45	6	42e	47	53	54	75	77	83a	84	85	81	94	96
Patient 1												±	±	++	++	++				++			
Patient 2												±	±	++	++	++				++			
Patient 3												±	±	++	++	++				++			
Surgeon												±	±	++	++	++				++			
Nurse	++		±									++	++			±			++	+			
Ward staff	±													+									

Fig. 19.2 Phage typing of *S. aureus*.

19 Questions

1 How would you investigate these wound infections?
2 What is the principle of phage typing?

1 It is important to determine if the three wound infections are epidemiologically connected and if so, what the source of infection was. Superficial infection of the wound occurring after some days, and most likely after the first dressing change, is more in favour of ward-associated sepsis. A deep wound infection occurring within 2 days of operation in patients who were operated on by the same surgical team, or on the same list or in the same theatre is more in favour of a theatre source of infection. The aim of the investigation is to establish a common factor between the three patients, which involves determining: (a) which theatre they were operated in; (b) the position on the operating list; (c) the members of the surgical team; (d) the date of operation; (e) type of operation; (f) date of onset of infection; and (g) occurrence of any other cases that may be linked to the three under investigation.

The antibiotic sensitivity of the isolates may be helpful in determining if there is any link between the patients. If the antibiotic sensitivities are very different, then it is unlikely that they are part of an outbreak.

Postoperative wound infections caused by different organisms may be due to a breakdown in sterile technique, either on the ward or in the theatre. In this case one should check-up on operative theatre or ward procedures, for example, how are dressing changes performed? Also, if the infections seem to have been acquired in the operating theatre, then was there any special event during the period of their operations, such as too many people in the operating theatre? Additionally, the quality of the theatre air should be checked by sampling and the engineers consulted about ventilation maintenance.

The bacteria should be sent to a reference laboratory for typing. In this case of wound infections caused by *S. aureus*, phage typing is the most appropriate typing method.

If the *S. aureus* strains from the three patients can be distinguished from one another by phage typing, then this has the same implications as if the antibiotic sensitivity had been different. If, on the other hand, the strains are indistinguishable, this implies a single source of infection. This is usually a carrier of the epidemic strain who is on the ward or working in theatres. Screening swabs should be taken from all staff members who have had contact with the three patients. Nose and/or groin swabs are taken and any *S. aureus* isolated sent to the reference laboratory for phage typing to determine if they are indistinguishable from the bacteria isolated from the index cases.

In this case, the phage-typing pattern of the three patients and an isolate from the surgeon are the same and the isolates are regarded as indistinguishable. These isolates have a different phage pattern from strains isolated from a theatre nurse or ward staff. The source of this outbreak can be traced to the surgeon. The surgeon should be excluded from theatre and put on an eradication protocol to eliminate staphylococcal carriage. An eradication protocol consists of the application of antistaphylococcal nasal cream and shampoo and total bathing in an antistaphylococcal medication for 1 week. This is followed by rescreening the carrier sites for persistence of the organism.

2 When a bacterium is infected with a bacteriophage, most of the bacteria lyse but a small proportion become lysogenic, where the bacteriophage is integrated into the bacterial chromosome as a prophage. Bacteria that are lysogenized by a particular bacteriophage are resistant to superinfection (and thus lysis) by the same bacteriophage.

In phage typing of S. aureus, an internationally agreed set of different bacteriophages is spotted onto a culture of S. aureus that has been spread over the surface of an agar plate. The bacteriophage are spotted onto the S. aureus culture at a routine test dilution (RTD) and at 100 times the RTD. The agar plate is then incubated and the following day the pattern of lysis is inspected. The lysis is recorded as + + or − (Fig. 19.2). If the three S. aureus cultures from the three patients have the same pattern of lysis, they are reported as indistinguishable and if there is epidemiological evidence linking infection in the three patients, the laboratory data are supportive evidence of cross-infection or, in this case, a single source of infection.

References

Bengtsson S, Hambraeus A & Laurell G (1979) Wound infection after surgery in a modern operating suite: clinical bacteriological and epidemiological findings. *J. Hyg. Camb.* **83**, 41–56.

Glenister HM, Taylor LJ, Bartlett CLR, Cooke EM, Sedguick JA & Mackintosh CA (1993) An evaluation of surveillance methods for detecting infections in hospital inpatients. *J. Hosp. Infect.* **23**, 229–242.

A young girl developed a spreading annular scaly lesion on her arm. Skin scrapings were taken for culture (Fig. 20.1). The organism took 2 weeks to grow after which a preparation of the growth was examined microscopically (Fig. 20.2).

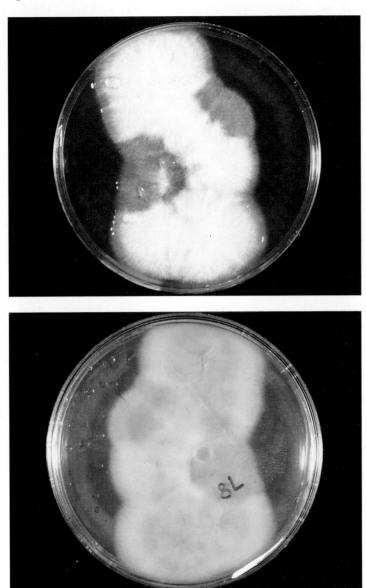

Fig. 20.1

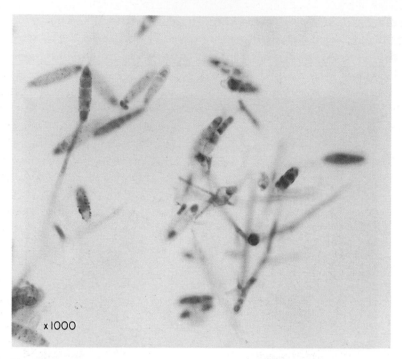

x 1000

Fig. 20.2

Questions
1 What is your diagnosis?
2 What are the sources and routes of transmission of this organism?
3 How should the girl be treated?

Answers

1 Clinically the lesion could be ringworm (tinea corporis). Skin scraping from the lesion viewed directly would show fungal elements present in the skin. The skin scrapings are also inoculated onto agar. Fungi that colonize the keratinized epithelium of the skin (dermatophytes) take 1–2 weeks to grow (Fig. 20.1). The type of dermatophyte is identified from the macroscopic characteristics of the culture (colour and texture of the growth) and by macroscopic examination of the culture (Fig. 20.2). There are principally three genera of dermatophytes. *Trichophyton*, *Microsporum*, *Epidermophyton* and many species have characteristically shaped macrosporidia (spores). The fungus shown here is *Microsporum*.

Dermatophytes can infect various regions of the body, including the hair, producing the clinical conditions tinea cruris and tinea capitis. Other superficial fungal skin infections are white piedra (*Trichosporum beigelii*) and black piedra (*Piedraia hortea*), which produce white or black nodules upon the hair and lead to alopecia; and tinea versicolor (*Malassezia furfur*), which produces pigmented or depigmented patches on the skin, exacerbated by sunlight.

2 Ringworm may follow inoculation of spores into the superficial layers of the skin. Most species of ringworm are restricted to humans (anthropophilic) and infection occurs mostly by indirect contact from an infected person to a non-infected person via contaminated fomites, for example, combs, razors, shower floor—e.g. *Tinea rubrum*. Direct person-to-person contact may also spread anthropophilic dermatophytes. Some species of dermatophytes are spread from infected animals to humans, for example, *Microsporum canis*, and some infections are derived from contact with contaminated soil, for example, *M. gypseum*.

3 Lesions of limited extent, particularly if inflamed, can often be treated successfully with topical agents, such as undecenoic acid or miconazole.

Extensive lesions, particularly if chronically inflamed, should be treated with oral griseofulvin or oral ketoconazole.

References

Finch R (1988) Skin and soft tissue infections. *Lancet* **1**, 164–167.
Jones HE (1982) Therapy of superficial fungal infections. *Med. Clin. North Am.* **64**, 873–893.

21 The air in an operating theatre was sampled during a total hip replacement operation (Fig. 21.1). The number of bacteria-carrying particles (BCP) per cubic metre of air was 150. A Gram stain of the colonies (Fig. 21.2) and a slide coagulase test were performed (Fig. 21.3).

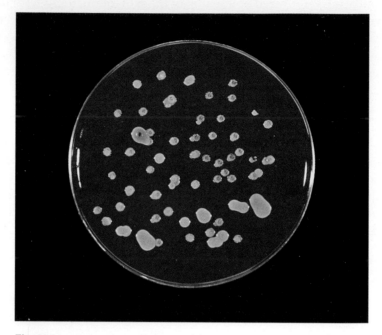

Fig. 21.1

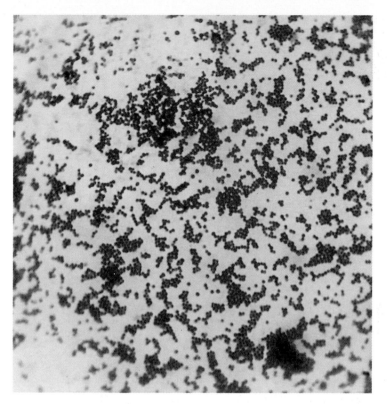

Fig. 21.2

21

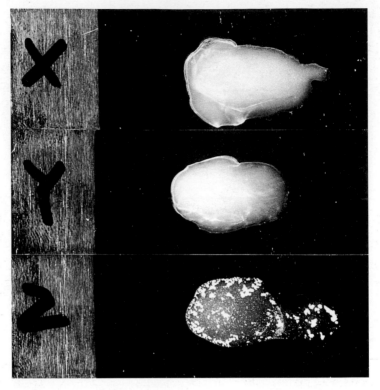

Fig. 21.3 X, test: organism isolated from theatre air; Y, slide coagulation test negative; Z, slide coagulation test positive.

Questions

1 What is the identity of the organism?
2 What is its origin?
3 Is the count in the air excessive for this type of operation? If so, how can it be reduced?

Answers

1 The organism is a coagulase-negative staphylococcus (CNS). This is because the Gram stain shows it to be a Gram-positive coccus arranged in clusters, and the organism does not cause clumping of plasma when mixed together on a slide. The identity of the organism would be confirmed by biochemical tests. Without these tests, it would not be possible to differentiate staphylococci from other Gram-positive cocci arranged in clusters that may also be found in the air, such as micrococci.

   There are many different species of CNS. The one most frequently causing infections is *Staphylococcus epidermidis*. Other important CNS are *S. saprophyticus*, causing urinary tract infections in females, and *S. lugdenensis*, which can cause skin infections and endocarditis on otherwise healthy heart valves. *S. epidermidis* causes prosthetic valve endocarditis, urinary tract infections associated with catheters, peritonitis associated with chronic ambulatory peritoneal dialysis, septicaemias associated with infected venous access lines, such as Hickmann lines, and infected orthopaedic prostheses, such as hip replacements.

2 The organism originated from the people in the operating theatre. All people desquamate 10^3 BCP/min. These particles are skin scales, colonized by the commensal flora of the skin, which are sloughed off, particularly during movement and friction against clothes. Females tend to desquamate more than males and desquamation occurs mainly from below the waist. Some individuals desquamate at a much higher rate than the average and they are called dispersers. About 10% of males compared to 1% of females are dispersers. The mean size of the skin scales is 14 μm and they sediment out of the air at an average rate of 0.3 m/min.

3 The number of BCP in the air depends upon the number of individuals, the movement and the presence of any dispersers. In a conventionally ventilated operating theatre with 20 changes of air per hour, 150 BCP would be an acceptable bioload. In orthopaedic operations involving a prosthesis, this is too high a bacterial count because the chance of the patient developing an infected prosthesis is high. For this type of operation the BCP should not be greater than $10/m^3$. This value can be achieved by restricting the number of people in theatre and using an ultraclean air ventilation system, in which filtered air is directed over

21   the operating table, giving 200 air changes per hour; the operating team are dressed in theatre clothes and gowns made of bacteria-impenetrable material.

References

Hambraeus A (1988) Aerobiology in the operating room: a review. *J. Hosp. Infect.* **11** (Suppl. A), 68–76.

Lidwell OM, Lowbury EJL, Whyte W, Blowers R, Stanley SJ & Lowe D (1982) Effect of ultraclean air in operating rooms on deep sepsis in the joint after total hip or knee replacements: a randomised study. *Br. Med. J.* **285**, 10–15.

A 3-year-old child developed a high temperature and was complaining of earache. On examination the ear drum was bulging and erythematous. A myringotomy was performed and the pus sent to the laboratory for microscopy (Fig. 22.1) and culture.

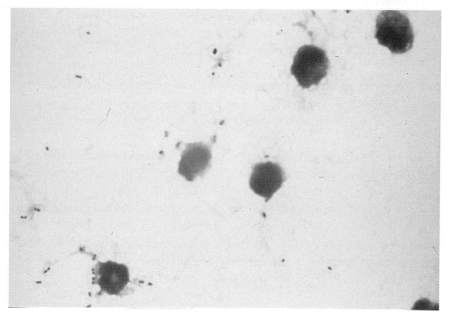

Fig. 22.1

Questions
1 What are the common causes of this condition? Which organism is present here?
2 How should the patient be treated?
3 What complications may occur?

Answers

1 Otitis media can be caused by viruses or bacteria and it is not possible to distinguish clinically between them. The most common bacterial causes of this condition are *Streptococcus pneumoniae* (seen in Fig. 22.1) and *Haemophilus influenzae*. Other bacterial causes are *Staphylococcus aureus* and *Streptococcus pyogenes*. *Mycoplasma pneumoniae* can be a rare cause of myringitis. Both the *S. pneumoniae* and *H. influenzae* causing otitis media are often acapsulate varieties.

2 The patient should be given amoxycillin. Alternative antibiotics that can be used are co-amoxiclav (if a β-lactamase-producing organism is the cause, e.g. β-lactamase-positive *H. influenzae*) or co-trimoxazole.

3 Perforation of the ear drum may occur. The infection may spread to produce mastoiditis, a cerebral abscess or meningitis. The condition may become chronic otitis media, where the middle ear becomes superinfected with Gram-negative bacteria, for example, *Proteus*, and anaerobic bacteria, for example, *Bacteroides*. A sterile effusion may follow acute otitis media and this is called glue ear. Hearing loss may supervene either acute otitis media or glue ear.

Reference

Brook I (1994) Microbiology and management of bacterial respiratory tract infections. *Rev. Med. Microbiol.* **5**, 3–11.

A lawyer who 3 days previously had returned from abroad presented at 23 a casualty department complaining of a sore throat, orodynia, headache and general malaise. He was pyrexial and had a tachycardia. On examination of the pharynx a firmly adherent membrane was seen on the fauces. A swab was taken and sent to the microbiology department for microscopy (Fig. 23.1) and culture (Fig. 23.2). Also in the laboratory a test was performed on the isolate, the results of which are shown in Fig. 23.3.

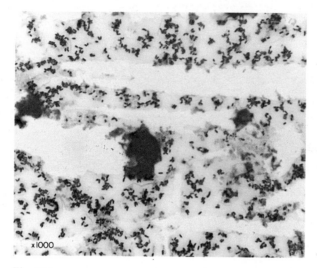

Fig. 23.1

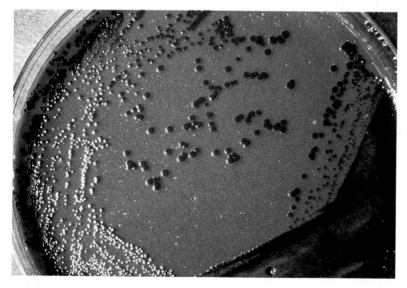

Fig. 23.2

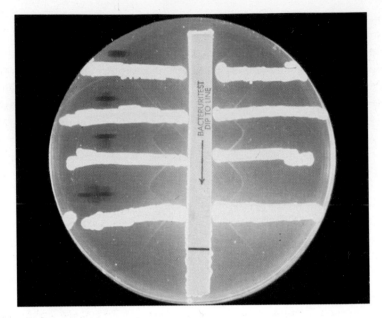

Fig. 23.3

Questions
1 What complications may follow this infection? How is the illness caused?
2 How is the diagnosis confirmed microbiologically? What is the test shown in Fig. 23.3?
3 How may his illness be prevented and how should the patient be managed?

Answers

1 Clinically the patient has diphtheria. This is an illness caused by toxigenic strains of *Corynebacterium diphtheriae*. It can also rarely be caused by toxigenic strains of other corynebacteria—*C. ulcerans*. Toxigenic strains are lysogenized by a bacteriophage which carries the information coding for the toxin. The organism is transmitted by droplet infection and has an incubation period of 2–7 days. Diphtheria can present with the bacteria infecting different regions of the upper respiratory tract—nasopharynx, fauces, larynx—producing a characteristic firmly adherent membrane. Alternatively, the patient may present with one of the toxin-induced complications of the illness without any prominent evidence of local nasopharyngeal infection. Diphtheria may also follow cutaneous infection with a toxigen strain. This occurs most frequently in tropical countries and the patient has a sharply defined, punched-out skin ulcer. Only sporadic cases of diphtheria occur in the UK, but large epidemics have occurred in other countries, such as Russia.

Strains of *C. diphtheriae* that are lysogenized by the β-bacteriophage produce an exotoxin which diffuses from the site of local infection in the nasopharynx into the blood. The toxin is composed of two subunits: one binds to receptors on cell members and facilitates the entry of the other subunit into the cytoplasm of the cell. This subunit is an enzyme with adenosine diphosphate (ADP) ribosylating activity and transfers ADP-ribose from nicotinamide adenine dinucleotide (NAD) to elongation factor 2 (EF2), an important protein necessary for the normal functioning of ribosomes during protein synthesis. The effect of the toxin is to inactivate EF2 and stop protein synthesis in affected cells.

Local complications can follow infection, with laryngeal obstruction caused by an extensive membrane, or oedema of the neck, which leads to a bull-neck appearance and respiratory embarrassment. Diphtheria may present with evidence of cardiovascular, neurological or renal damage caused by the action of the toxin on cranial, cardiac or peripheral nerves or the cells of the renal tubules. Cardiovascular toxicity may be evident, with paralysis of respiration, palatial paralysis, diplopia or paralysis of a limb; albuminuria indicates damage to renal cells.

2 A throat and nose swab should be taken for microscopy and culture. The swabs are plated onto a selective, differential medium (Hoyle's or Tinsdale's medium) and an enrichment medium (Loeffler's slope).

23 Suspect colonies are identified biochemically and the production of toxin is detected by Elek's method (Fig. 23.2). A filter paper soaked in antitoxin is placed on an agar plate and the suspect organism is inoculated at right angles, with appropriate positive and negative controls. The agar plate is incubated and toxin production by the isolate is detected by looking for an easily visible line indicating immune complex toxin–antitoxin precipitation. The isolate should be sent to the reference laboratory for confirmation. Polymerase chain reaction (PCR) may replace the Elek method for detecting toxigenic isolates.

3 Once a clinical diagnosis of diphtheria has been made and a throat and nose swab taken for microbiology, the patient should be nursed in source isolation, preferably in an infectious diseases unit. The patient should be given antitoxin and started on erythromycin. The disease is notifiable and the consultant in communicable diseases should be informed. A list of contacts should be prepared, to include domestic, social and occupational contacts, as well as health care staff who have seen the patient. Nose and throat swabs should be taken from all contacts and close contacts should be given erythromycin as chemoprophylaxis. Asymptomatic carriers of toxigenic *C. diphtheriae* and secondary cases should be isolated, treated as the index case and further contacts sought.

The disease may be prevented by vaccination using a preparation of formaldehyde-inactivated toxin, called a toxoid, which is combined with an adjuvant, such as aluminium hydroxide. Primary vaccination is given along with tetanus and pertussis vaccines at 2, 3 and 4 months of age, with a booster dose at 5 years. Absorbed low-dose diphtheria vaccine may be given to adults either as a booster or as a primary course, depending on their previous immunization record.

Reference

Barksdale L, Garmise L & Horibata K (1960) Virulence, toxigenicity and lysogeny in *Corynebacterium diphtheriae. Ann. N.Y. Acad. Sci.* **88**, 1093–1108.

A young child presented at a casualty department acutely ill with stridor. An emergency tracheostomy was performed. The patient was pyrexial and blood cultures were taken (Fig. 24.1). The organism's dependence upon X and V factors was determined (Fig. 24.2).

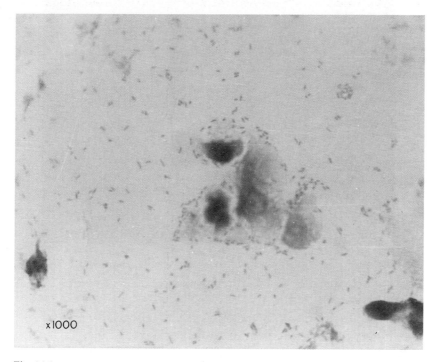

x1000

Fig. 24.1

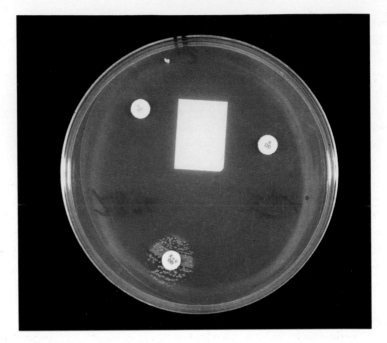

Fig. 24.2

Questions
1 What is your clinical and microbiological diagnosis?
2 What other illnesses does this organism cause?

Answers

1 The patient has epiglottitis. The organism causing this is *Haemophilus influenzae*. It is a slender Gram-negative bacillus that is nutritionally dependent upon both X (haemin) and V (nicotinamide adenine dinucleotide—NAD) factors, as shown by growth only around the disc containing both factors. Growth around the V-containing discs would indicate *H. parainfluenzae* and growth around the X-containing discs would indicate *H. ducreyi*.

2 Apart from epiglottitis, other severe invasive disease may occur with *H. influenzae*, such as orbital cellulitis, meningitis, pyogenic arthritis and osteomyelitis. *H. influenzae* biotype III (*H. aegyptius*) causes a severe infection in children characterized by petechiae and hypotension, called Brazilian purpuric fever. Non-capsulate *H. influenzae* are a cause of sinusitis, otitis media or exacerbations of chronic bronchitis along with *Streptococcus pneumoniae*, and can occur at any age.

References

Heney C, Berkowitz F, Baise T *et al.* (1990) Spread of non-typable multiply resistant *H. influenzae* in a South African hospital. *Eur. J. Clin. Microbiol. Infect. Dis.* **9**, 24–29.

Turk DC (1984) The pathogenicity of *H. influenzae*. *J. Med. Microbiol.* **18**, 1–18.

25 A patient with AIDS presented with dysphagia. Examination of the oropharynx showed areas of reddened mucosa. On oesophagoscopy, thick white plaques were seen, which were swabbed and a Gram stain prepared (Fig. 25.1).

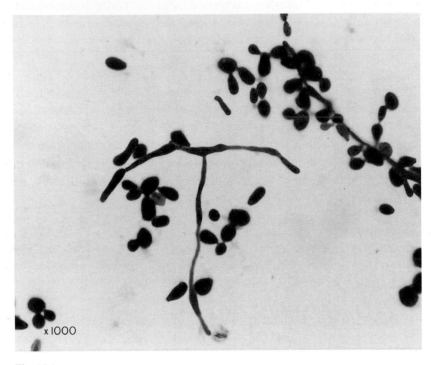

x 1000

Fig. 25.1

Questions

1 What is your diagnosis? How is this confirmed microbiologically?
2 Which other infections can give this clinical picture in AIDS patients?
3 What is the treatment?

1 The swab of the oesophageal plaques shows the presence of a yeast, with the typical oval morphology, presence of budding forms and hyphae. The patient has oral and oesophageal candidiasis. Oral candidiasis does not always present, as in this case, with areas of red-dened mucosa. Dysphagia is a common symptom of oesophageal candidiasis.

The swab should be plated onto Sabouraud's medium and in-cubated. Colonies of yeast will grow in 24–48 h, which can then be identified by a combination of biochemical and mycological analysis.

In addition to producing oro-oesophageal infection in AIDS patients, *Candida* can cause systemic infection in other immuno-compromised patients. Candidaemia may be complicated by endophthalmitis or endocarditis. Other predisposing factors for *Candida* infections are the use of broad-spectrum antibiotics and dia-betic ketoacidosis. Specific T-cell defects may lead to a chronic mucocutaneous infection. Infection may complicate chronic ambu-latory peritoneal dialysis, giving peritonitis, and systemic infection may occur in patients receiving total parenteral nutrition. Local infections can occur in the mouth and vagina (thrush) and *Candida* may infect areas of macerated skin – intertrigo, paronychia.

2 The other main cause of dysphagia in AIDS patients is ulceration of the oesophagus, caused principally by cytomegalovirus.

3 This patient should be treated with fluconazole initially and if the patient does not respond to adequate doses, the treatment can be changed to parenteral amphotericin. Superficial infections in the oropharynx may respond to nystatin or amphotericin lozenges.

Amphotericin and nystatin are both polyenes. Their mode of action is to produce a transmembrane pore in the cytoplasmic membrane of the fungus, through which intracellular components are lost. They both bind to ergosterol in the fungal membrane. Because of the similarity of the fungal cytoplasmic membrane to human cytoplasmic membranes, the polyenes also bind to the human cell membrane and are there-fore toxic. Nystatin cannot be given parenterally because of this. Amphotericin can be given parenterally, although it is nephrotoxic. The nephrotoxicity can be reduced by giving liposomal amphotericin – amphotericin encapsulated in a lipid micelle.

Antifungal azole compounds act by inhibiting carbon-14 α-sterol demethylation and thus the synthesis of ergosterol. Currently, the antifungal azoles are: clotrimazole and miconazole, which are usually used as topical agents for superficial *Candida* infections; and ketoconazole, fluconazole and itraconazole, all of which can be given orally, which are used for systemic infections, like cryptococcal meningitis. Itraconazole has activity against *Aspergillus* and can be used for invasive pulmonary aspergillosis.

References

Bodey GP (1992) Azole antifungal agents. *Clin. Infect. Dis.* **14** (Suppl. 1), S161–S169.

Lec W, Burnie JP, Matthews RC, Oppenheim BO & Damain NN (1991) Hospital outbreaks with yeasts. *J. Hosp. Infect.* **18** (Suppl. A), 237–249.

A civil engineer returning from India developed acute watery diarrhoea on arrival at Heathrow. Over a period of 24 h he became rapidly dehydrated because of the diarrhoea. A specimen of the liquid faeces was plated onto thiosulphate citrate bile salt sucrose (TCBSS) agar and incubated (Fig. 26.1).

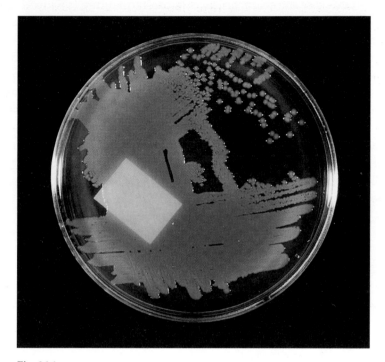

Fig. 26.1

Questions
1 What is your clinical suspicion and how should you confirm it?
2 What is the mechanism of pathogenesis of his illness?
3 What public health implication does this case have?

26 Answers

1 The clinical suspicion with this history would be of cholera.

The rapid dehydration is a consequence of massive loss of water and electrolytes in the liquid 'rice-water' faeces. The specimen should be placed onto one of the selective differential media, such as TCBSS agar. In this case the characteristic sucrose-fermenting (yellow) colonies of *Vibrio cholerae* are seen. These have to be confirmed as *V. cholerae* by biochemical and serological testing of the isolate. There are many different species of *Vibrio* and they are naturally found in coastal and river water. Some can cause superficial skin infections following bathing in coastal waters; some are associated with gastroenteritis linked to consumption of shellfish (*V. parahaemolyticus*) and *V. cholerae* causes the clinical illness cholera. The species, *V. cholerae*, can be subdivided into serotypes—01, 02, etc. Cholera is caused by *V. cholerae* serotype 01 and, more recently, *V. cholerae* serotype 0139, a novel, hitherto unrecognized cholera serotype. The other serotypes of *V. cholerae* can cause gastroenteritis but clinically it is not as severe as cholera. *V. cholerae* 01 can be further sero- and biotyped. Outbreaks of cholera have occurred with the classical biotype, which was replaced by the El Tor biotype and this seems as if it is being replaced as the epidemic cholera strain by *V. cholerae* 0139 (Bengal).

2 Cholera toxin is a multicomponent protein with five subunits involved in binding of the toxin to receptors on gastrointestinal cells. These subunits aid the entry of the active subunit into the cytoplasm of the cell, where it affects the regulatory protein of the adenyl cyclase enzyme, which is found on the basolateral membrane of gastrointestinal epithelial cells. This inhibition results in an increase in cAMP levels in the cell which ultimately leads to a massive loss of water and electrolytes from the gastrointestinal tract, principally the small intestine.

3 Cholera is spread where there is poor sanitation. A case of cholera entering the UK does not pose a threat to public water supplies because of the water treatment by the supply utilities. This patient should be source-isolated, rehydrated and given tetracycline. The consultant in communicable disease should be notified.

A vaccine comprising heat-killed organism can be given to travellers to endemic areas. The protection is short-lived and is not very effective (about 50%).

References

Bhattacharya SK, Bhattacharya MK, Balakrish Nair G *et al.* (1993) Clinical profile of acute diarrhoea cases infected with the new epidemic strain of *V. cholerae* 0139: designation of the disease as cholera. *J. Infect.* **27**, 11–15.

Deb BC, Bhattacharya SK & Pal SC (1990) Epidemiology of cholera in India and its treatment and control. *Curr. Sci.* **59**, 702–707.

27 Upper gastrointestinal endoscopy was performed on a patient who had been complaining of epigastric abdominal pain and who subsequently presented with a haematemesis. At endoscopy a duodenal ulcer was seen. Gastric biopsies were taken for a rapid urease test (Fig. 27.1), histology (Fig. 27.2) and culture.

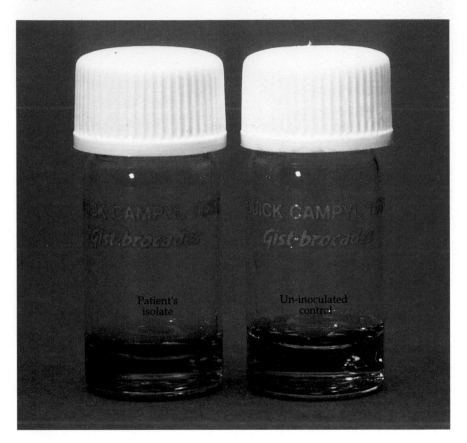

Fig. 27.1

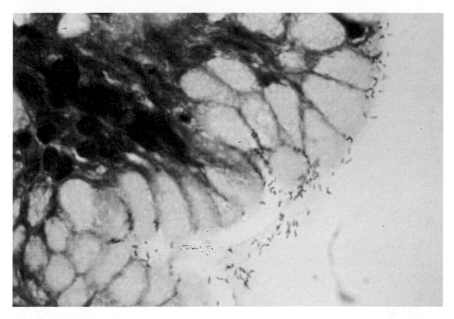

Fig. 27.2

Questions
1 What is the organism that is present in the stomach?
2 What is the rapid urease test?
3 What relationship does the organism have to the ulcer?
4 How should the patient be managed?

27 Answers

1 The organism is *Helicobacter pylori*. This is a curved microaerophilic bacterium that is found attached to the epithelial layer of gastric mucosa where it causes inflammation. The organism is transmitted from person-to-person, probably by the faecal–oral route, although epidemiological evidence suggests that contaminated water supplies may also act as a source of infection. In western Europe and the USA there is an increasing seroprevalence with increasing age, such that by the age of 60 years, 50% of individuals are colonized by the organism. In Africa and Asia as many as 80% of the population can be colonized by the age of 5 years. Colonization of the stomach inevitably results in inflammation, although in most cases this is asymptomatic.

2 Because *H. pylori* takes 5 days to produce visible colonies on agar, more rapid tests are used to detect it. *Helicobacter* characteristically produces an abundant amount of urease enzyme which hydrolyses urea to produce carbon dioxide (CO_2) and ammonia. This can be used as a diagnostic marker for the presence of *H. pylori*. At endoscopy a biopsy of the stomach is taken and placed in an unbuffered solution of urea with a pH indicator. The hydrolysis of the urea to produce ammonia changes the pH indicator. A positive test can be obtained within 5 min. The presence of *H. pylori* can also be determined by culture or histology examination of the biopsy specimen. Colonization by *H. pylori* can also be detected without endoscopy, by either a serological test to detect anti-*H. pylori* antibodies or the urea breath test. In this latter test carbon-13 (^{13}C)- or ^{14}C-labelled urea is given to the patient as a test meal and the evolution of $^{13}CO_2$ or $^{14}CO_2$ in the breath can be determined, indicating the presence of *H. pylori* in the stomach.

3 *H. pylori* causes peptic ulceration. The fact that only a relatively small proportion of individuals who are colonized by *H. pylori* go on to develop ulceration indicates that other factors are involved. Certain strains of *H. pylori* are ulcerogenic and variation in the virulence properties of the organism would seem to be an important consideration. The mechanisms of pathogenesis are not yet clear, although several potential ones are recognized. Some strains of *H. pylori* produce a cytotoxin and all strains produce ammonia, caused by the action of its urease enzyme. The presence of the organism in the stomach may lead to antibodies cross-reacting with gastric epithelium and causing damage to the cells. *H. pylori* induces a hypergastrinaemia and hyperpepsinogenaemia, which leads to excess acid and pepsin in the stomach. Finally, the protective mucous barrier in the stomach is affected by the presence of the organism.

The relationship between *H. pylori* and non-ulcer dyspepsia (NUD) is controversial, although there is evidence suggesting that some patients with NUD do have symptomatic improvement when the organism is eradicated.

Long-term colonization by *H. pylori* is a significant risk factor for the development of gastric cancer. *H. pylori* is also the cause of low-grade gastric B-cell lymphoma.

4 *H. pylori* can be eradicated from the stomach by the use of a combination of bismuth + metronidazole + amoxycillin or tetracycline given for 2–4 weeks. An alternative regimen that is of current interest is a combination of omeprazole and either amoxycillin or clarithromycin given for 2 weeks. Eradication rates of 90% can be achieved and in those patients with duodenal ulceration the ulcer relapse rate is very much reduced (less than 5%) if the organism is successfully eradicated.

Reference

Vaira D, Holton J, Miglioli M, Menegatti M, Mulé P & Barabara L (1994) Peptic ulcer disease and *Helicobacter pylori* infections. *Curr. Opin. Gastroenterol.* **10**, 98–104.

28 Shortly after returning from Africa, a patient became unwell with a cough, temperature and constipation. Several days later the patient's condition deteriorated and he developed diarrhoea. He was admitted to hospital where on examination he was noted to have a rash and splenomegaly. His white blood cell (WBC) count was $4.0 \times 10^9/l$. A blood culture was taken (Fig. 28.1) and his faeces were cultured (Fig. 28.2).

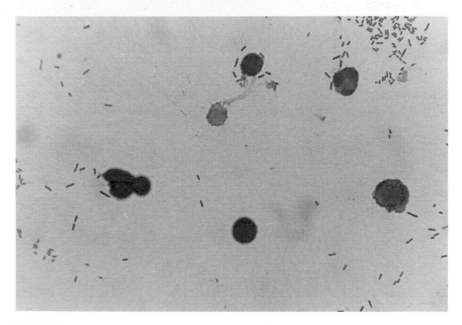

Fig. 28.1

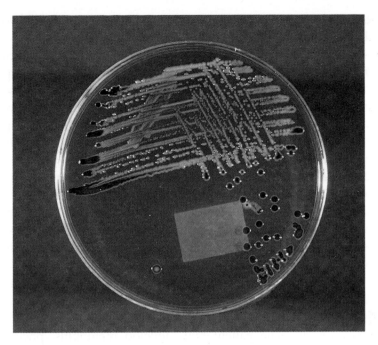

Fig. 28.2

Questions

1 What is your provisional diagnosis?
2 How would you confirm it bacteriologically?
3 How should the patient be treated?

29 Five children presented with fever, abdominal pain and diarrhoea streaked with blood, over a period of 3 days. They all attended the same primary school. Upon investigation by the environmental health department, it was found that one of the children had recently been abroad on holiday with its family, two members of which also had abdominal pain and diarrhoea with blood in the faeces. Faecal specimens were collected and inoculated onto deoxycholate citrate agar (DCA) medium. A non-lactose-fermenting organism was present which failed to agglutinate with *Salmonella* polyvalent O antisera and was subsequently tested with *Shigella* antisera (Fig. 29.1). The results were confirmed by biochemical testing of the isolate.

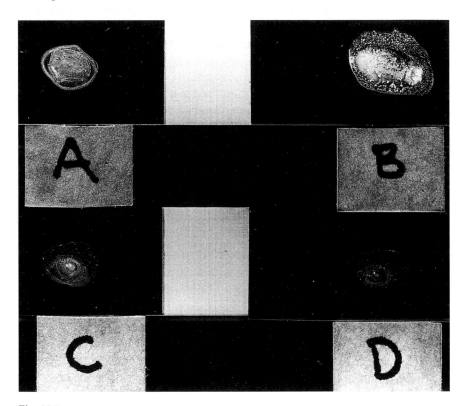

Fig. 29.1

Questions

1 What is the identity of the organism?
2 What is the mode of spread?
3 What systemic complication may occur with this infection:
   (a) *Shigella dysenteriae*?
   (b) *S. flexneri*?
   (c) *S. boydii*?
   (d) *S. sonnei*?

29 Answers

1 *S. flexneri*. DCA contains bile and is inhibiting to many of the commensal flora of the intestine. It also contains lactose and a pH indicator, which allows one to distinguish between organisms that ferment lactose (producing red colonies) and organisms that do not ferment lactose (producing pale-coloured colonies).

A small number of bacterial species that can be found in the faeces of people, such as *Pseudomonas* and *Proteus*, do not ferment lactose and these are distinguished from *Salmonella* and *Shigella* which are also non-lactose-fermenting, by biochemical tests. The serological tests are performed by emulsifying the organism with specific antisera; the presence of agglutination (Fig. 29.1) indicates the identity of the organism. Because the structure of the cell walls of enteric bacteria is very similar, serological cross-reactions may occur and therefore the biochemical reactions of the organism are determined in addition to the agglutination tests. In this case agglutination has occured with *S. flexneri*.

There are four species of *Shigella*: *S. dysenteriae*, *S. flexneri*, *S. boydii* and *S. sonnei*. *S. sonnei* is the species most commonly isolated in the UK and it is frequently associated with a mild attack of dysentery. The other species give a much more severe attack of dysentery and are usually imported into the UK by travellers, as in this case.

2 The main route of infection is direct person-to-person spread by the faecal–oral route, or from contaminated objects, such as door handles. Spread is facilitated by poor hygienic conditions, when hand-washing facilities in lavatories are not present or are not used. Outbreaks of dysentery may occur in institutions, like schools, where the requirement for hand-washing after going to the lavatory may not be appreciated. In contrast to *Salmonella*, only a few organisms (about 100) are required to initiate an infection and the incubation period is 1–2 days before symptoms develop. In some countries contaminated food or water may act as a source of infection and *Shigella* may be transmitted by flies. Dysentery is a notifiable disease in the UK. Outbreaks in schools are controlled by excluding the symptomatic cases, reinforcing the importance of hand-washing and disinfection of lavatory facilities.

3 *Shigella* multiply locally in the colonic epithelial cells, producing necrotic ulcers and giving rise to the symptoms of bloody diarrhoea. Painful swollen joints—knees and ankles—may occur 1–2 weeks following an attack of dysentery. This is a reactive arthritis and can be caused

by other gastrointestinal infections, for example, *Campylobacter* or
Yersinia.

Dysentery caused by *S. dysenteriae* may be complicated by the haemolytic–uraemic syndrome.

Patients should not be given antibiotics, as the majority of cases are mild, particularly if caused by *S. sonnei*. In severe cases, ciprofloxacin, co-trimoxazole or ampicillin can be given in addition to fluid replacement.

References

Levine OS & Levine MM (1991) Horseflies as mechanical vectors of shigellosis. *Rev. Infect. Dis.* **13**, 688–696.

Pickering LK, Bartlett AV & Woodward WE (1986) Acute infectious diarrhoea among children in day care: epidemiology and control. *Rev. Infect. Dis.* **8**, 539–547.

30 Twenty-four hours after attending a convention, a patient became ill with a temperature, abdominal pain, vomiting and diarrhoea. Faeces were collected and inoculated onto selective differential media and into selenite F broth. Colonies suspected of being *Salmonella* (Fig. 30.1) were identified biochemically (Fig. 30.2) and serologically and phage-typed. The organism was finally identified as *Salmonella enteritidis* phage type 4.

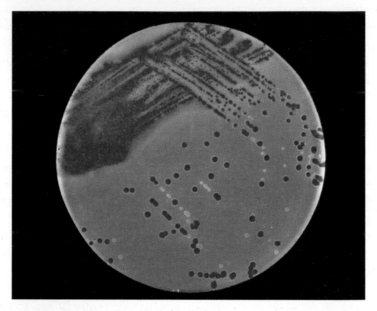

Fig. 30.1

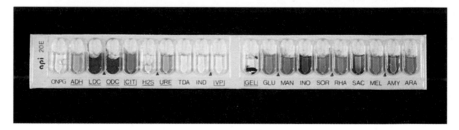

Fig. 30.2

Questions
1 Which colonies should be investigated further?
2 How should this patient be managed?
3 What is the food likely to cause this infection?
4 What are the steps involved in making a bacteriological diagnosis of an enteric infection from the faecal specimen?

1 The pale-coloured colonies are non-lactose-fermenting organisms. *Salmonella* and *Shigella* are both non-lactose-fermenting and therefore it is these colonies that should be investigated. This is done by performing preliminary biochemical screening to exclude *Proteus* and *Pseudomonas*, which are also non-lactose-fermenting and which produce pale-coloured colonies on this medium.

2 Antibiotics have no role to play in the management of the majority of cases of *Salmonella* gastroenteritis. Exceptions are if the gastroenteritis occurs in an individual who is immunocompromised or if there is evidence of systemic invasion in any patient. Dehydration and electrolyte imbalance should be corrected by fluid replacement. Control of the diarrhoea by drugs is contraindicated because of the risk of inducing paralytic ileus and causing septicaemia.

   Food poisoning, as this case would seem to be from the history, is a notifiable condition and should be reported to the consultant in communicable disease control. Because the patient has attended a convention, it is very likely that she is part of an outbreak and all persons attending the convention should be contacted to find out if they have been symptomatic and to collect faecal specimens for culture. Specimens of food, if still available, should also be collected for culture.

3 *S. enteritidis* phage type 4 has been epidemiologically linked to the use of contaminated hens' eggs.

4 It is important that clinical information concerning the patient is given to the laboratory. Faeces from the patients who present with enteric infections are inoculated onto selective or selective and differential media and the type of media used depends upon the clinical circumstances and the suspected pathogen.

   All faeces are routinely inoculated onto a selective differential medium, for example, McConkey's medium or deoxycholate citrate agar (DCA), and into selenite enrichment broth (selenite F). Additional media would be used if clinically indicated, for example, the use of thiosulphate citrate bile salt sucrose (TCBSS) agar if cholera was suspected. The selective differential media used is a preliminary screening procedure in order to pick out bacteria that could be enteric pathogens. In this case, *Salmonella* does not ferment lactose and grows in the presence of bile (which inhibits most of the commensal microflora). Pale colonies (Fig. 30.1; non-lactose-fermenting organisms) are therefore picked off for more detailed biochemical and serological testing.

Different bacteria have characteristic patterns of biochemical reactions (Fig. 30.2) and these can be tested most conveniently in commercially produced galleries of test, with different test galleries comprising different sets of biochemical reactions appropriate for the major groups of bacteria. The series of biochemical reactions shown in Fig. 30.2 is appropriate for enteric organisms, the coliforms, which include both *Salmonella* and *Shigella*, are two important enteric pathogens.

There are about 1500 species of *Salmonella*, which are mainly differentiated serologically. The cell wall of *Salmonella* (and other coliforms) is antigenic and is called O antigen. If the organism is motile it will have flagellae, which are also antigenic and called H antigen. The various species of *Salmonella* have different combinations of O and H antigen. This serological scheme for identifying *Salmonella* is called the Kaufmann–White scheme.

The particular O and H antigen an isolate has, is determined by emulsifying a colony with specific, commercially produced antibodies on a glass slide. If agglutination (clumping) of the organism occurs with the different O and H antibodies, then the respective antigens are present on the isolate. For example, in this patient *S. enteritidis* was isolated, which has O antigens 1, 9 and 12 and H antigens g, m, 1 and 7. (The two series of O and H antigens both given numerals are quite separate types of antigens and not related to each other.)

Some species of *Salmonella* can be subdivided into phage types (the principle is the same as phage-typing of *Staphylococcus aureus*, except that a different set of bacteriophages is used). Typing is essential for epidemiological investigation of outbreaks and defining a common source for the infection.

Reference

Reid TMS (1992) The treatment of non typhi salmonellosis. *J. Antimicrob. Chemother.* **29**, 4–8.

A patient became unwell with fever and myalgia, which was followed 2 days later by acute cramping abdominal pain and diarrhoea, streaked with blood. Faeces inoculated onto deoxycholate citrate agar (DCA) medium yielded only lactose-fermenting colonies but when inoculated onto a selective medium and incubated under microaerobic conditions yielded a heavy growth of an organism (Fig. 31.1). A Gram stain was performed from the colonies on the selective medium (Fig. 31.2).

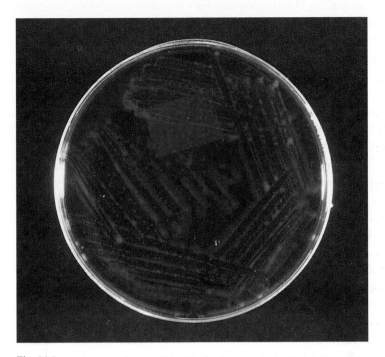

Fig. 31.1

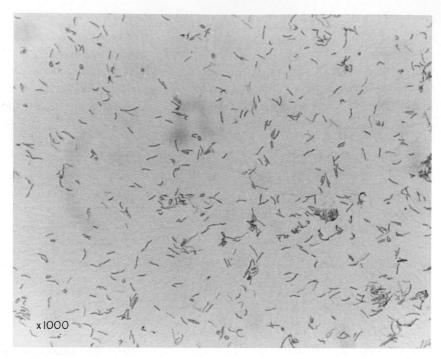

Fig. 31.2

Questions

1 What is the presumptive identity of the organism?
2 What is the management of the patient?
3 What neurological complication may follow this infection?

Answers

1 The organism is *Campylobacter jejuni*. Enteric infections with this organism may often be preceded by systemic symptoms of headache, malaise and myalgia. Abdominal pain is often severe and cramping, and blood is frequently mixed in with the faeces. The organism is not detected on DCA medium. Selective medium containing antibiotics is used and the specimen is incubated under microaerobic conditions. Colonies are visible within 48 h (Fig. 31.1) and are confirmed as *Campylobacter* by a Gram stain (Fig. 31.2) and biochemical tests.

   The main source of infection is from poultry, although contaminated milk has also been a vehicle for outbreaks. Infection may be acquired from symptomatic dogs. Long-term faecal carriage is unusual. *Campylobacter* is the commonest bacterial cause of gastroenteritis in the UK.

   Many species of *Campylobacter* exist apart from *C. jejuni*, some of which also cause gastroenteritis. *C. coli* is particularly likely to give a septicaemic illness.

2 Most patients do not require treatment, but with severe symptoms, erythromycin can be used. An alternative effective antibiotic is ciprofloxacin.

3 Reactive arthritis may follow *Campylobacter* enteritis. Rarely, the haemolytic–uraemic syndrome occurs. From 1 to 6 weeks following enteritis, a polyneuropathy may develop – the Guillain–Barré syndrome. Although not a common complication, because *Campylobacter* enteritis is a common infection, up to 30% of cases of Guillain–Barré syndrome give a history of having had *Campylobacter* enteritis in the preceding 6 weeks. The pathogenesis of the illness is probably linked to an antibody against a component of the bacterial cell wall, cross-reacting with a component of the nerve cell.

References

Konkel ME, Mead DJ & Cieplak W (1993) Kinetic and antigenic characterisation of altered protein synthesis by *Campylobacter jejuni* cultivated with human epithelial cells. *J. Infect. Dis.* **168**, 948–954.

Penner JL (1988) The genus Campylobacter: a decade of progress. *Clin. Microbiol. Rev.* **1**, 157–172.

A 15-year-old was admitted to hospital with right lower quadrant abdominal pain and tenderness. A diagnosis of appendicitis was made and the patient operated upon. The appendix was normal but the mesenteric lymph nodes were enlarged. On further questioning, it was found that his 4-year-old brother had had an episode of diarrhoea with a temperature and abdominal pain which resolved spontaneously; the father, who had also complained of gastroenteritis, had subsequently developed swollen and painful ankles and knees and red painful nodules on his shins. A non-lactose-fermenting Gram-negative organism that grew on a selective medium (cefsulodin–Igrasan–novobiocin medium) was isolated from the mesenteric lymph node in the 15-year-old and from the faeces of the 4-year-old.

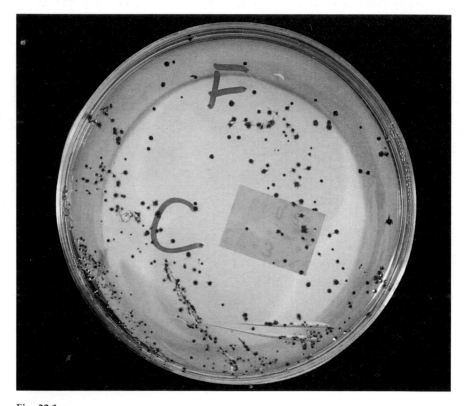

Fig. 32.1

Questions

1 What is your provisional identification of the organism?
2 Is the father's illness related to that of his children?
3 What treatment would you advise?

1 The provisional identity of the organism is *Yersinia*, either *enterocolitica* or *pseudotuberculosis*. These organisms produce characteristic colonies on this selective medium (Fig. 32.1). The clinical history is suggestive of yersiniosis.

2 Yes, the father's illness is likely to be related to an infection with the same organism as that affecting his children. The presentation of yersiniosis differs depending upon the age of the patient. In the younger age group an infection presents as gastroenteritis or mesenteric adenitis. In adults infection may be followed by extraintestinal systemic manifestations such as reactive arthropathy and erythema nodosum. The illness may also present as generalized lymphadenopathy or septicaemia and chronic infection can present as a fever with abscesses in liver and spleen.

Y. enterocolitica is only occasionally isolated from the faeces. The organism may be isolated from lymph nodes. The usual method of diagnosis of yersiniosis is by serology, although in chronic infection, serum agglutinins and culture may both be negative. In these cases diagnosis can be made by immunoblotting against *Yersinia* outer membrane proteins.

3 Gastroenteritis is self-limiting and does not usually require antibiotics. Evidence of systemic illness or chronic yersiniosis will respond to doxycycline or co-trimoxazole.

References
Cover TL & Aker RC (1989) *Yersinia enterocolitica. N. Engl. J. Med.* **321**, 16–24.
Hoogkamp-Korstanje JAA (1987) Antibiotics in *Yersinia enterocolitica* infections. *J. Antimicrob. Chemother.* **20**, 123–131.

33 A 56-year-old woman was operated upon for diverticulitis and whilst on the ward was given a cephalosporin for a presumed chest infection. Several days after starting the antibiotics, the patient became unwell with severe abdominal pain and blood-stained diarrhoea. A faecal sample was sent to the laboratory for testing; the results are shown in Fig. 33.1.

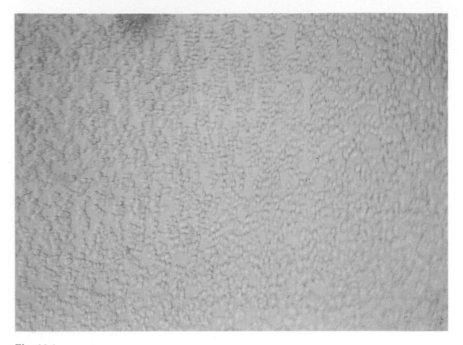

Fig. 33.1

Questions
1 What is the likely diagnosis?
2 What is the test shown in Fig. 33.1?
3 How is the infection transmitted?
4 How should the patient be treated?

1 Severe abdominal pain and blood-stained diarrhoea in a patient who is on antibiotics should always raise the suspicion of pseudomembranous colitis (PMC). The diagnosis is confirmed by sigmoidoscopy where characteristic lesions are seen on the colon wall. In some cases lesions may be produced higher up in the gastrointestinal tract beyond the range of the sigmoidoscope. Occasionally, patients will present with abdominal pain with minimal diarrhoea. The diagnosis can be confirmed in the laboratory by the detection of the cytotoxin in the faeces.

2 A monolayer of cells is exposed to the faeces and the characteristic cytopathic changes, of cells rounding up, looked for after a period of incubation. Figure 33.1 demonstrates the cytopathic effect due to exposure of the monolayer to a faecal extract. It is also possible to isolate the causative organism, *Clostridium difficile*, from the faeces on selective media. The prevalence of faecal carriage is low in adults but can be as high as 35% in neonates in the absence of symptoms.

3 The organism is disseminated into the environment from an index case and can be recovered from floors and bed-frames. Outbreaks of hospital-acquired infection have been reported and a patient who has *C. difficile*-associated diarrhoea should be isolated. The laboratory detection of toxins has a high positive predictive value for disease. PMC may occur several weeks after finishing a course of antibiotics.

4 Antibiotics should be stopped. In many cases, if the patient does not have PMC, the diarrhoea stops. If PMC is confirmed the patient should be given either oral vancomycin or metronidazole for 14 days. Relapses are common and a further course of treatment may be required. Alternative treatment can be with cholestyramine (which binds the toxin) or re-establishment of the normal flora by oral *Saccharomyces boulardis* or an enema of human faeces.

References

Pothoulakis C, Castagliuolo I, Kelly CP & Lamont T (1993) *Clostridium difficile*-associated diarrhoea and colitis: pathogenesis and therapy. *Int. J. Antimicrob. Agents* **3**, 17–32.

Fekety R, Kim KH & Brown D (1981) Epidemiology of antibiotic associated colitis. Isolation of *C. difficile* from the hospital environment. *Am. J. Med.* **70**, 906–908.

34 Three children were admitted to hospital over a period of 2 days with diarrhoea followed by anaemia and thrombocytopenia, and progressing to renal failure. Cultures of faeces were sent to the microbiology laboratory, where *Escherichia coli* was isolated (Fig. 34.1).

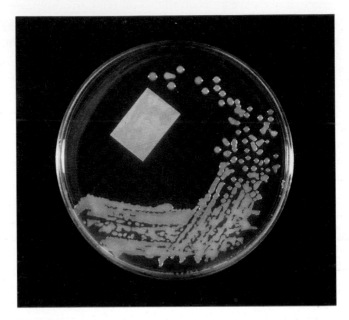

Fig. 34.1

Questions

1 What illness do the children have?
2 Of what relevance is the isolation of *E. coli*? What further characterization of the isolate is required?
3 What epidemiological implications does this incident have?
4 With what other gastrointestinal illnesses is *E. coli* associated?

1 The children have the haemolytic–uraemic syndrome (HUS), which is a combination of microangiopathic thrombocytopenia, haemolytic anaemia and renal failure.

2 The cause of HUS is a Verotoxin-producing strain of *E. coli*. The toxin is very similar to the Shiga toxin produced by strains of *Shigella dysenteriae* type 1. Two types of Verotoxin can be produced by *E. coli*−one whose effect can be neutralized by Shiga antitoxin, and one that cannot (VT1 and VT2, respectively). The toxins consist of two subunits, the B subunit mediating binding to cells and the A subunit responsible for cytotoxicity.

    Verotoxin-producing strains of *E. coli* belong mainly to one serotype, O157, H7 and characteristically do not ferment sorbitol. Sorbitol-negative colonies can be detected on a differential medium (Fig. 34.1) and the serotype determined by slide agglutination tests with antisera to the cell wall O antigen 157 and the flagella, H antigen 7. Verotoxin production can be confirmed by detecting a cytopathic effect upon Vero cell monolayers, which can be neutralized with antitoxin. Verotoxin-producing strain in faeces may also be detected by colony hybridization using a DNA probe. The toxin may be detected directly in the faeces.

    In addition to causing the HUS, *E. coli* O157 also causes a haemorrhagic colitis (which may be followed by HUS).

3 Outbreaks of both clinical conditions have been reported and food is often a common source, for example, undercooked hamburgers. In this case the three children may be part of a larger outbreak and should be reported to the consultant for communicable disease control.

4 *E. coli* produces a number of other gastrointestinal illnesses.

    Enteropathogenic *E. coli* (EPEC) is a cause of infantile gastroenteritis and the strains belong on a number of different serotypes. The mechanism of pathogenesis is unclear but *E. coli* attach to mucosal cells, producing an 'adhesion pedestal' in response to the presence of the bacteria.

    Some strains of *E. coli* produce toxins, in addition to the Verotoxin mentioned above. These strains are called enterotoxigenic *E. coli* (ETEC) and produce either heat-labile toxin (LT) or heat-stable toxin (ST). LT is structurally similar to cholera toxin and has a similar mode of action,

34   increasing intracellular cAMP. ST is a low-molecular-weight peptide, which increases intracellular cyclic guanosine monophosphate (cGMP). ETEC is a prominent cause of traveller's diarrhoea.

Enteroadhesive or aggressive strains of *E. coli* (EAEC) are an additional cause of gastroenteritis and like EPEC adhere to enterocytes, but with marked loss of microvilli on the mucosal cell.

Enteroinvasive *E. coli* (EIEC) is a further group associated with diarrhoeal illness. This group invades enterocytes and induces cell death with tissue destruction. In this respect they are similar to *Shigella*.

References

Karmali MA, Petric M, Lim C, Fleming PC, Arbus GS & Lior H (1985) The association between idiopathic haemolytic uraemic syndrome and infection by Verotoxin-producing *E. coli. J. Infect. Dis.* **151**, 775–782.

Ratnam S, March SB, Ahmed R, Bezanson G & Kasatiya S (1988) Characterisation of *E. coli* serotype O157:H7. *J. Clin. Microbiol.* **26**, 2006–2012.

A young woman was admitted to hospital complaining of rigors and loin pain and a diagnosis of pyelonephritis was made. A midstream specimen of urine was taken and sent to the laboratory for investigation. The results of the culture (Fig. 35.1) and the sensitivities (Fig. 35.2) are shown.

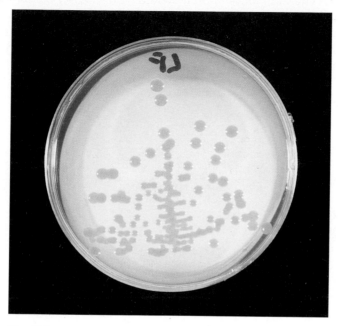

Fig. 35.1

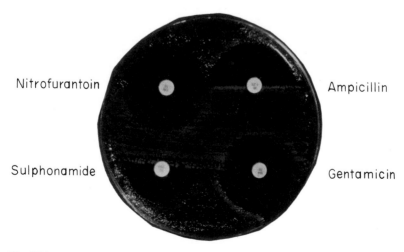

Fig. 35.2

35 Questions

1 What is the most likely identity of the organism?
2 What bacterial factors are involved in the pathogenesis of this bacterial infection?
3 Which of the antibiotics shown would you choose, based upon the sensitivities shown in Fig. 35.2?

1 The organism most frequently causing pylonephritis is *Escherichia coli* (60–80% of cases). Other important bacterial causes of urinary tract infection are *Proteus*, *Klebsiella* and *Pseudomonas* (which is particularly common in hospital-acquired urinary infection, compared to community-acquired infection); *Enterococcus faecalis* and *Staphylococcus saprophyticus* (which is particularly associated with community-acquired infection in young females).

   Midstream specimens of urine are plated onto a differential medium (cysteine lactose electrolyte-deficient – CLED). The specimen should be processed quickly after collection because a semiquantitative assessment of the number of organisms per millilitre of urine is performed, by plating out a standard volume of urine. If there is a delay before specimen processing, the relative proportions and absolute numbers of different bacteria may change, which may give a false impression of their importance. Patients who have pylonephritis are more likely to have a single species of bacterium in amounts greater than 10^5 cfu/ml (equivalent to greater than 100 colonies growing on the medium). In this case the patient has more than 100 colonies of one type – the colonies look morphologically identical. As the medium contains lactose and a pH indicator it is possible to determine if the organism ferments lactose, producing yellow colonies (*E. coli*, as in this case), or does not ferment lactose by producing pale colonies, such as *Proteus* or *Pseudomonas*. The identity of the organism is confirmed by testing its biochemical reaction and sensitivities are performed (Fig. 35.2). A number of different commercially produced automated machines may be used to screen specimens of urine for those which contain a significant bacteriuria (greater than 10^5 cfu/ml).

2 The source of *E. coli* in cases of pyelonephritis is the faecal flora and infection occurs in an ascending fashion, with bacteria contaminating the perineum colonizing the urethra and bladder and vesicoureteric reflux infecting the kidneys.

   Strains of *E. coli* which cause pyelonephritis possess a number of virulence factors. One important factor is the presence of bacterial *P. fimbriae* which mediate adherence to uroepithelial cells, particularly which have P blood group specificity (α D gal 1-4β D gal). Other virulence factors associated with *E. coli* strain causing pyelonephritis are the production of a haemolysin and the possession of a plasmid (called CoIV because it carries information-producing colicines which are antibacterial substances) carrying the genetic information for the production of aerobactin (an iron-binding protein which transports iron into the bacterial cell).

Other virulence properties of E. coli, not linked to pyelonephritis, are toxin production, whether heat-labile toxin (LT), heat-stable toxin (ST) or Verotoxin, linked to gastroenteritis; fimbrial adhesions (complement-fixing antibody (CFA) I–IV) present in enterotoxigenic E. coli (ETEC) strains also linked to gastroenteritis and capsular antigens, for example, K1, the possession of which is associated with E. coli that cause neonatal meningitis.

3 The sensitivities of this isolate have been determined by disc diffusion using the Stokes method. In this method a bacterial strain acting as a control is plated across the outer sectors of the agar. The control organism is known to be sensitive to the antibiotics used. The patient isolate is spread across the middle of the plate and filter-paper discs containing antibiotic are placed at the junction between the control organism on the patient's isolate. During incubation the antibiotic diffuses out into the medium, inhibiting the growth of sensitive bacteria around the antibiotic-containing discs. If a zone of inhibition of the patient's isolates is equal to or greater than the zone of inhibition of the control, the patient's isolate is sensitive to the antibodies. If the zone of inhibition of the patient's isolate is less than that of the control, the patient's isolate is resistant.

In this case the E. coli is sensitive to nitrofurantoin acid and gentamicin but resistant to trimethoprim and amplicillin. Because it is necessary to use an antibiotic that achieves tissue penetration to treat pyelonephritis, then, of the four antibiotics shown here, gentamicin would be the antibiotic chosen. Nitrofurantoin may be used for cystitis but not pyelonephritis, as it does not achieve sufficient serum levels to inhibit the organism.

References

Kallenius G, Mollby R, Suensai SB et al. (1981) Occurrence of P-fimbriated E. coli in urinary tract infections. Lancet 2, 1369–1372.

Krogfelt KA (1991) Bacterial adhesion: genetics biogenesis and role in pathogenesis of fimbrial adhesions of E. coli. Dev. Infect. Dis. 13, 721–735.

A middle-aged male patient complained of a sharp pain in his loin radiating down to his perineum, accompanied by haematuria. A midstream specimen of urine was collected for culture and sensitivities. The results of the culture on cysteine lactose electrolyte-deficient (CLED) medium (Fig. 36.1) and on blood agar (Fig. 36.2) are shown. The organism was identified biochemically as *Proteus*.

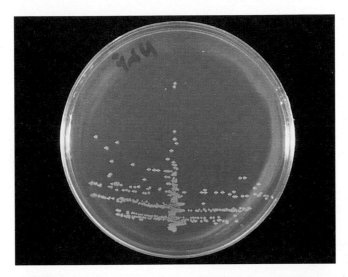

Fig. 36.1

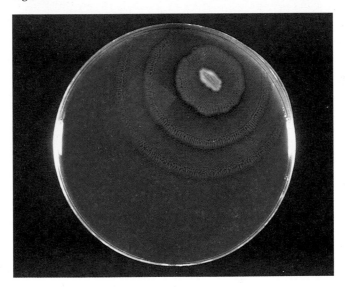

Fig. 36.2

Questions

1 What is your clinical suspicion about the cause of the patient's symptoms and how may it be confirmed?
2 What relevance may the isolation of the *Proteus* have to his illness?

Answers

1 Clinically the history is that of renal colic caused by passing renal stones. The patient may give a history of passing renal stones during micturition. A plain abdominal X-ray may reveal renal stones and the patient needs an intravenous urogram.

2 The organism isolated is a *Proteus*. Biochemically this produces a urease enzyme which hydrolyses urea. The hydrolysis of urea produces ammonia which makes the urine alkaline. It is under these conditions that calcium and phosphates will precipitate to produce renal stones.

   Also note from Fig. 36.1 the usefulness of CLED medium in inhibiting the swarming of *Proteus*. On blood agar (Fig. 36.2) *Proteus* will swarm over the plate, obscuring colonies of other organisms that could be present. This swarming is inhibited on CLED medium.

References

Andriole VT (1987) Urinary tract infections: recent developments. *J. Infect. Dis.* **156**, 865–869.

Kraiden S, Fuksa M, Lizewski W, Barton L & Lee A (1984) *Proteus penneri* and urinary calculi formation. *J. Clin. Mircobiol.* **19**, 541–542.

37 A paraplegic patient, with a long-term urinary catheter, had a urine specimen sent for routine culture. The results of the culture are shown in Fig. 37.1.

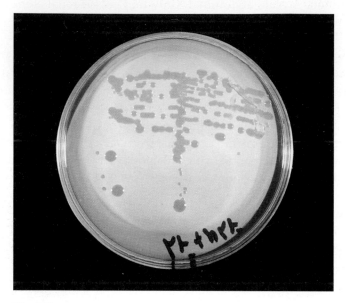

Fig. 37.1

Question
1 What is your interpretation of the microbiology results and what action would you take?

1 The culture is mixed, including a non-lactose-fermenting organism (the pale colonies). This is probably a *Pseudomonas* species, which is commonly found colonizing urinary drainage systems.

The relevance of the finding depends upon the patient's clinical state. If the patient is asymptomatic then the findings may be of no immediate relevance, although a urinary tract colonized by bacteria can act as a focus of infection. Antibiotics should not be given because, although they may temporarily suppress the bacteria, as soon as they are stopped recolonization will occur as long as the catheter is in place. Also, giving antibiotics may select for an antibiotic-resistant organism. This is more difficult to treat if the patient should subsequently become septicaemic. If the patient is symptomatic, with a pyrexia, a blood culture should be taken and the appropriate treatment started, depending upon the sensitivities of the organism isolated. If possible the catheter should be removed, although in some instances this is not a practical proposition.

References

Bodey GP, Bolivar R, Fainsteom V & Jadeja L (1983) Infections caused by *P. aeruginosa. Med. Infect. Dis.* **5**, 279–311.

Claytar CL, Chaula JC & Stichler DJ (1982) Some observations on urinary tract infections in patients undergoing long term bladder catheterization. *J. Hosp. Infect.* **3**, 39–47.

38 A female patient presented with dysuria and a vaginal discharge. A midstream specimen of urine yielded a mixed growth of less than 10^5 cfu/ml bacteria. An endocervical specimen was taken for microscopy (Fig. 38.1) and culture.

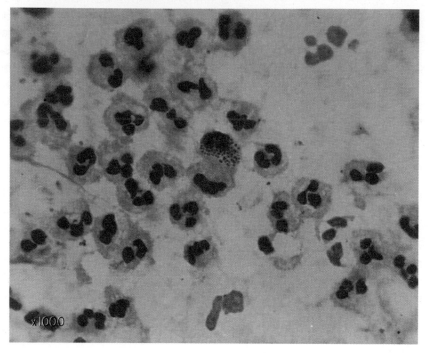

Fig. 38.1

Questions
1 What is your diagnosis?
2 What complications are associated with this infection?
3 How should the patient be managed?

1 The patient has gonorrhoea. The slide shows intracellular Gram-negative diplococci, which are *Neisseria gonorrhoeae*. The microscopic findings would be confirmed by culture and biochemical identification of the isolate.

   N. gonorrhoeae is an organism susceptible to adverse environmental conditions. In practice, an endocervical swab must be taken (rather than a high vaginal swab), plated onto a selective medium and incubated immediately in an atmosphere containing 5% carbon dioxide at 37°C. The same applies to a male patient, except a urethral swab is taken. The sensitivity and specificity of microscopy in the female are much lower than in the male, where gonorrhoea can be diagnosed with a high degree of certainty by microscopy. In both sexes, however, the diagnosis must be confirmed by culture.

2 Female patients are more likely to have asymptomatic infections than male patients. In addition to genital infections, anorectal, pharyngeal and conjunctival infections occur. Endocervical infections in pregnant females can lead to abortion and premature rupture of membranes. A neonate born to an infected mother may have conjunctival infection— ophthalmia neonatorum. In females pelvic inflammatory disease and perihepatitis may follow endocervical infection and in males, prostatitis or epididymitis may occur. Systemic infections may occur, most commonly septic arthritis, although rarely endocarditis, osteomyelitis or meningitis have been reported.

3 The patient should be treated with oral amoxycillin and probenecid. The probenecid reduces the renal excretion of the β-lactam.

   If the isolate produces a β-lactamase, an injection of ceftriaxone or oral ciprofloxacin can be used.

   In patients who have systemic complications such as pelvic inflammatory disease, in which *N. gonorrhoeae* is isolated, a 10-day course of ampicillin or parenteral penicillin is required.

   The patient should be followed up after initial treatment in order to monitor eradication of the organism. It is essential that the patient's contacts are sought and appropriate specimens taken from them.

38 Reference

Britigan BE, Cohen MS & Sparling PF (1985) Gonococcal infection: a model of molecular pathogenesis. *N. Engl. J. Med.* **312**, 1683–1692.

A male patient presented with a urethral discharge and dysuria. A speci- men of the urethral discharge was collected for microscopy and culture for *Neisseria gonorrhoeae*, both of which were negative. A specimen was sent for culture of *Chlamydia trachomatis*. The results are shown in Fig. 39.1.

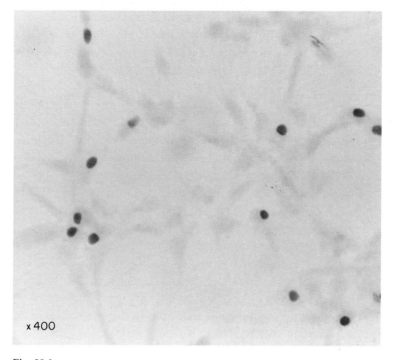

x 400

Fig. 39.1

Questions
1 How was the specimen processed and what does it show?
2 What other illnesses are carried by *Chlamydia*?
3 How should the patient be managed?

39 Answers

1 The specimen is sedimented onto a monolayer of cyclohexamide-treated fibroblasts (McCoy cells) and incubated for 2–3 days. The monolayer is then stained with iodine, which detects the glycogen-containing inclusions produced by the growth of *C. trachomatis*. In addition to staining with iodine, growth can be confirmed by direct immunofluorescent staining for *Chlamydia*.

   C. trachomatis may be rapidly detected in some specimens by the use of labelled antibodies to chlamydial antigen.

2 *C. trachomatis* can be divided into three biogroups corresponding to serogroups A–C, D–K and L_1–L_3. *C. trachomatis* A–C causes trachoma, a chronic keratoconjunctivitis, which is endemic in tropical countries and a major cause of blindness. *C. trachomatis* D–K causes non-gonococcal genital infections, as in this case, in both males and females. In the female the *Chlamydia* are detected in the endocervix and may be associated with pelvic inflammatory disease and perihepatitis. This biogroup causes acute conjunctivitis in adults and in neonates born to infected mothers. The organism can also cause a pneumonia in neonates between 4 and 12 weeks of age. *C. trachomatis* L_1–L_3 causes lympho-granuloma venereum, which presents with genital ulceration and regional lymphadenopathy, which, with time, may suppurate.

   C. psittaci causes a number of infections in different animals, including birds, which act as a source of infection for humans. In humans, *C. psittaci* causes a pneumonia which can vary between a mild flu-like illness to a severe pneumonia with rash and splenomegaly.

   C. pneumoniae causes a respiratory flu-like illness and has been responsible for large outbreaks of infection in Scandinavia and the USA. The illness is characterized by pharyngitis and myalgia; hoarseness is a common feature.

3 The patient should be treated with tetracycline for at least a week. Contact tracing of the patient's sexual partners is mandatory, as it is for gonorrhoea, in order to eradicate effectively a community source of infections.

References
Ridgway GL (1993) The domiciliary management of genital tract infections. *J. Antimicrob. Chemother.* **32** (Suppl. A), 11–16.
Ridgway GL (1992) Advances in the antimicrobial therapy of chalmydial genital infections. *J. Infect.* **25** (Suppl. 1), 51–59.

A male patient presented at a dermatology department with a history 40
of malaise and a scaling, papular rash on the palms of his hands and an
ulcer on his hard palate. Further examination revealed a generalized non-
tender lymphadenopathy. Dark ground microscopy of scrapings of the
mucous ulcer revealed the organisms shown in Fig. 40.1.

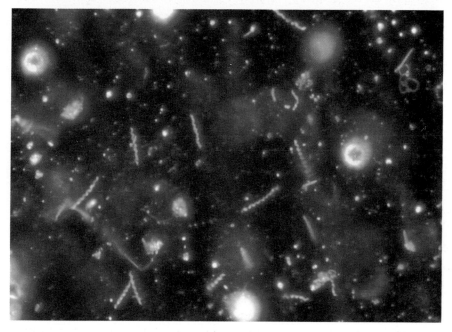

Fig. 40.1

Questions
1 What is your clinical suspicion of the diagnosis?
2 What further investigations would you perform?
3 How would you manage the patient?

1 The clinical presentation is suggestive of secondary syphilis and the dark ground microscopy of the ulcer scrapings shows spirochaetes consistent with *Treponema pallidum*.

    The primary clinical indication of syphilis is a painless ulcer, usually on the genitals, which develops about a month after infection. This is the chancre and may last for 6 weeks. The secondary stage is evident about 2 months after the chancre appears and presents with systemic manifestations of fever and malaise. A rash can be present which may be macular, papular or pustular, and is characteristically found on the palms of the hands and the soles of the feet as well as the trunk. Generalized lymphadenopathy is present and typical snail-track ulcers may develop in the mouth. The patient may also have hepatitis, iritis, papular growths around the genitals (condylomata lata) and alopecia. *T. pallidum* can be detected in scrapings of the chancre, the oral ulcers and the condylomata by dark ground microscopy. The patient is highly infectious during these stages.

    After the primary and secondary stages the patient may become asymptomatic and enter a latency stage which can last for up to 20 years before the signs and symptoms of tertiary syphilis develop. Tertiary syphilis can present with neurological or cardiovascular complications or gumma (granulomata) in any part of the body, for example, skin or bone.

2 *T. pallidum* cannot be cultured. Laboratory diagnosis is by microscopy, as in this case, and serology. Serologically it is not possible to distinguish between syphilis, yaws and pinta (skin diseases caused by *Treponema* closely related to *T. pallidum*). The differentiation between these three conditions is clinical and positive treponemal serology should never be reported as indicating that the patient has syphilis.

    Two groups of serological tests exist: the non-specific tests using cardiolipin as antigen—venereal disease research laboratory (VDRL) and rapid plasma reagin (RPR)—and the specific tests using treponemal antigens—*T. pallidum* haemagglutination test (TPHA) and fluorescent *Treponema* antibody absorbed test (FTA-abs). The serological investigation of suspected syphilis relies on a screening test (VDRL or TPHA) followed by a confirmatory test if the screening test is positive. In early primary syphilis both tests may be negative but the FTA-abs is the first test to become reactive at about the third week of illness. In secondary syphilis both the TPHA and the FTA-abs are nearly always positive.

Both tests remain positive for life, even with successful treatment. The VDRL of IgM-FTa-abs may be used to monitor the success of treatment. This patient should have syphilis serology performed.

40

3 The patient should receive procaine penicillin. If he is hypersensitive to β-lactams, erythromycin or tetracycline can be used. The patient should be regularly monitored clinically and serologically and contacts traced.

Reference
Young H (1993) Syphilis: new diagnostic directions. *Int. J. STD AIDS* **3**, 391–413.

41 A patient presented with a history of weight loss, anaemia, general malaise and a fever over several weeks. On examination the patient had a cardiac murmur and splenomegaly and was noted to have splinter haemorrhages. The patient also had microscopic haematuria. Blood cultures were taken and grew the organism shown in Figs 41.1 and 41.2.

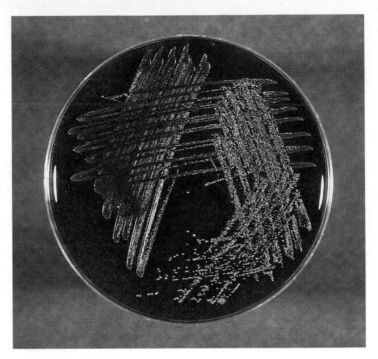

Fig. 41.1

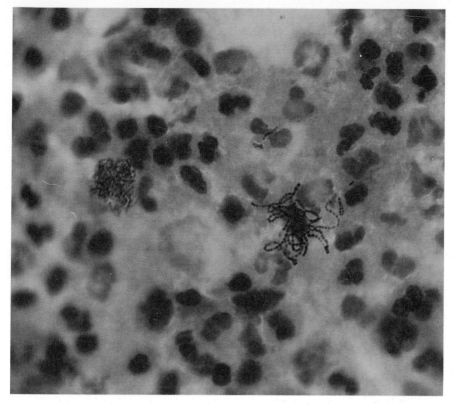

Fig. 41.2

Questions

1 What is your clinical diagnosis and what is the organism likely to be?
2 How should the patient be treated?
3 What other organism can cause this illness?

Answers

1 The patient has bacterial endocarditis. Often this is of insidious onset, as in this case, but it may present in an acute fashion with cardiac failure caused by valve rupture, or with central nervous system symptoms caused by embolic complications.

   The illness is caused by bacteria adhering to and multiplying on the valve leaflets. Usually, the endocardium is damaged by turbulent flow of blood, for example, a bicuspid valve, or some pre-existing condition which has damaged the heart valves, such as rheumatic fever. Occasionally, completely healthy valves can be colonized by some bacteria which cause endocarditis. The bacteria multiply on the heart valve, protected from host defence mechanism by fibrin and platelet aggregation which produce macroscopic vegetations within which the bacteria are located. The organisms may occasionally invade the vessel walls, producing an abscess. In addition to local damage to the heart valve, leading to regurgitation of blood and cardiac failure, systemic complications may occur, either immunologically mediated, such as nephritis caused by immunocomplex deposition in the kidneys, or by embolization of bits of the vegetation to other areas, for example, the central nervous system, causing focal neurological signs and symptoms.

   The most frequent cause of endocarditis is the viridans streptococci, as shown here. The organism is a Gram-positive coccus arranged in chains (streptococcus) and it produces α-haemolysis (a greenish appearance of the blood around the colonies—hence viridans) on blood agar. The viridans streptococci comprise several different species. Of the viridans group, the species most frequently causing endocarditis is *Streptococcus sanguis*. The natural habitat of these organisms is principally the oropharynx, forming part of the commensal microflora of this region.

2 If the streptococcus is sensitive to penicillin (a minimum inhibitory concentration (MIC) of less than 1.0 mg/l) the patient is treated with parenteral benzylpenicillin combined with gentamicin for 2 weeks followed by oral ampicillin and probenecid for a further 2 weeks.

   If the organism is less sensitive to penicillin (MIC greater than 1.0 mg/l) then benzylpenicillin and gentamicin should be given for 4 weeks followed by a further 2 weeks of ampicillin and probenecid. Depending upon the exact sensitivity and identity of the streptococcus, other antibiotic regimens are used, for example, other combinations of a β-lactam and an aminoglycoside, or a glycopeptide, with or without an aminoglycoside.

The MIC is the minimum amount of antibiotic that is required to inhibit the growth of the isolate. This is a laboratory test in which twofold dilutions of the antibiotic are made in broth, in a series of test tubes, and a standard inoculum of the streptococcus is added. After incubation, turbidity is looked for in each of the tubes, indicating growth of the organism. Starting with the highest dilution of antibiotic, the first tube that appears clear (i.e. no growth of the organism) contains the concentration of the antibiotic that is called the MIC.

3 Virtually every organism has been reported as a cause of endocarditis at least once. However, there are some organisms that are recognized to be frequent causes. The commonest cause are the viridans stretococci and included in this group are *Streptococcus bovis* and *Enterococcus faecalis*, whose natural habitat is the gastrointestinal tract rather than the oropharynx. *Staphylococcus aureus* is a frequent cause of endocarditis in drug addicts and affects principally the valves on the right side of the heart. Coagulase-negative staphylococci are important causes of endocarditis on prosthetic heart valves.

Reference
Editorial (1992) Chemoprophylaxis for infective endocarditis: faith, hope and charity challenged. *Lancet* **339**, 525–526.

42 A male patient presented at a casualty department complaining of vomiting and diarrhoea. The patient was pyrexial and hypotensive and was noted to have a boil on his forearm. A swab was taken from the lesion (Fig. 42.1). The organism was not isolated from the blood cultures. The patient was treated with appropriate antibiotics. Several days after admission the patient's skin began to desquamate, although his general condition improved.

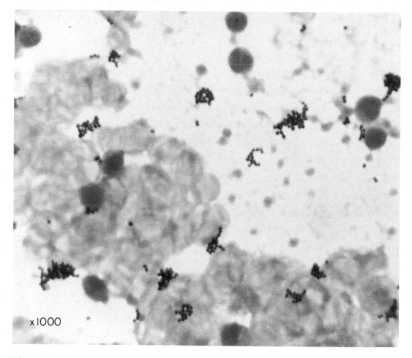

Fig. 42.1

Questions
1 What is the diagnosis and what is unusual about the presentation?
2 How is the illness caused?
3 What other similarly caused illnesses are associated with this organism?

Answers

1 The patient has toxic shock syndrome, characterized by fever, hypotension, vomiting, diarrhoea and skin desquamation. The unusual feature is that most cases of this illness occur in females. The condition was originally recognized in menstruating females, particularly if they were using a type of highly absorbent tampon. The cause of the illness is a *Staphylococcus aureus* that produces the toxic shock syndrome toxin TSST-1. A similar type of illness is also caused by *Streptococcus pyogenes*, which produces streptococcal pyrogenic exotoxins SPE A, B or C.

2 The toxin TSST-1 is a superantigen. This is a ligand which activates T cells by binding antigen-presenting cells, through a conserved sequence on the major histocompatibility complex (MHC) II receptor, to particular V_B chains of the T-cell receptor. Superantigens can activate 5–25% of the total T-cell population rather than the 1–2% activated by the more physiological mechanism of processed antigen at the MHC II site binding to both the α- and β-chains of the T-cell receptor. The pathophysiological effects of excessive release of cytokines leads to many of the signs and symptoms of the illness. Not all strains of *S. aureus* produce TSST-1.

3 *S. aureus* produces many different exotoxins in addition to TSST-1— exfoliating toxins ExT A and B, which cause the scalded skin syndrome; and enterotoxins Ent A–E, which cause food poisoning characterized by nausea and vomiting 1–5h after eating a meal contaminated by the preformed toxin. Both ExT A and Ent B are superantigens. In addition to the production of toxins with a characteristic clinical presentation, *S. aureus* produces a number of membrane-damaging toxins, cytolysins, and leucocidin, as well as other toxic products such as coagulase, staphylokinase and hyaluronidase.

References

Arbuthnott JP (1983) Host damage from bacterial toxins. *Phil. Trans. R. Soc. Lond. B* **303**, 149–165.
Zumla A (1992) Superantigens, T cells and microbes. *Clin. Infect. Dis.* **15**, 313–320.

43 A patient who was catheterized suddenly became pyrexial, acidotic, hypotensive and oliguric. A blood culture (Fig. 43.1) was taken. The same organism had previously been isolated from the urine; on biochemical testing it proved to be a *Klebsiella* species.

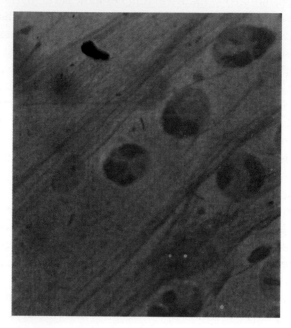

Fig. 43.1

Questions
1 What is the pathogenesis of this patient's condition?
2 Are antibiotics the correct choice to treat this condition?

Answers

43

1 The patient has septic shock caused by *Klebsiella* septicaemia. Gram-negative bacteria, such as *Klebsiella* or *Pseudomonas*, are frequently associated with colonization of the urinary tract in catheterized patients and this can act as a focus for the development of septicaemia. Septic shock can occur in about 40% of patients with septicaemia with either Gram-negative or Gram-positive organisms. A frequent cause of septicaemia, and therefore of septic shock, is *Escherichia coli*. The most potent inducer of septic shock is endotoxin, which is part of the cell wall of Gram-negative bacteria. The lipopolysaccharide present in the outer membrane of the cell wall of Gram-negative bacteria comprises a core region, which is similar in most Gram-negative bacteria, and a variable region of polysaccharides, which differs from one species of bacteria to the next. This lipopolysaccharide is the endotoxin; however, the principal biological activity resides in the core region which consists of a lipid moiety (lipid A) linked to a polysaccharide. Endotoxin originates a pathophysiological cascade of biochemical reactions by stimulating the production of a series of other factors which act as effectors. A pivotal role in septic shock is the lipopolysaccharide-induced production of tumour necrosis factor (TNF). Other cytokines, such as interleukin-1 (IL-1) and IL-6, and other factors, such as leukotriene, complement components and oxygen radicals, are produced at various points in the cascade of pathophysiological events, which ultimately result in tissue damage. The numerous effectors have a synergistic effect upon each other's production and action. The pathological end-result of this complex cascade of events is microvascular abnormalities caused by disseminated intravascular coagulation (DIC) and widespread tissue damage in many organs, with cell death. Septic shock has a mortality of about 75%.

2 Antibiotics should be given to patients with Gram-negative septicaemia although they make little difference to the outcome of established septic shock.

    An alternative approach to therapy is the use of antibodies directed against endotoxin or the mediators of septic shock, such as TNF. Immunotherapy for septic shock is still at a very early stage of development.

141

43 References

Bayston KF & Cohen J (1990) Bacterial endotoxin and current concepts in the diagnosis and treatment of endotoxaemia. *J. Med. Microbiol.* **31**, 73–83.

Stevens D, Bryant BS & Hackett SP (1993) Sepsis syndromes and toxic shock syndromes: concepts in pathogenesis and a perspective of future treatment strategies. *Curr. Opin. Infect. Dis.* **6**, 374–383.

Following an abdominal operation a patient became pyrexial and complained of right upper quadrant pain. Blood cultures were taken and an abdominal ultrasound scan was performed; this showed the presence of an abscess. The abscess was drained and the pus collected (Fig. 44.1). **44**

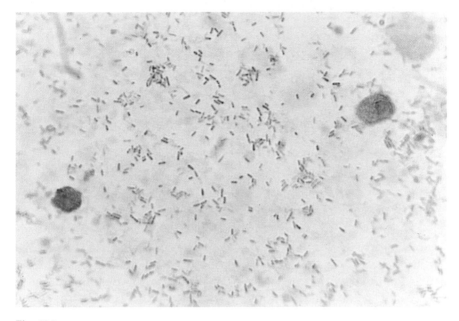

Fig. 44.1

Questions

1 What would you do with the pus and why?
2 What organisms are likely to be responsible for this intra-abdominal abscess, taking the results of microscopy into account?

44 Answers

1 The pus should of course be sent to the microbiology department, but despite the obviousness of this, all too frequently pus from an abscess is poured down the sluice and a swab, dipped in the pus, is sent to the microbiology department instead. Abscesses are often caused by anaerobic microorganisms that may not survive transport on a swab and in any case may take 48–72 h to grow on culture media. Pus is a very good transport medium and will keep anaerobes viable for a longer period of time than if sent on a swab. Also, the metabolic end-product of anaerobic metabolism, volatile fatty acid, can be detected by gas–liquid chromatography of the pus within a matter of a few hours. This investigation cannot be performed with a swab. The rapid detection of anaerobic organisms may modify the antibiotic treatment of the patient.

The treatment of an abscess is drainage, often combined with antibiotics. Metronidazole is the most appropriate antibiotic to use. Although reported, resistance to metronidazole is rare in *Bacteroides*.

Bacteroides fragilis does not respond to ampicillin, because the organism produces a β-lactamase. However, co-amoxiclav would be active because of the β-lactamase inhibitor (clavulanic acid) in the formulation. Benzylpencillin can be used for anaerobic infections. It is active against Gram-positive anaerobes, such as *Peptostreptococci* or *Clostridium*, but is not active against the Gram-negative *Bacteroides*. It is the antibiotic of choice for prophylaxis or treatment of gas gangrene.

Clindamycin has useful antianaerobic activity, particularly where mixed aerobic and anaerobic infections occur. It is as active as metronidazole against *B. fragilis*.

2 The organism seen on microscopy is a Gram-negative bacillus and therefore the most likely organism is *B. fragilis*. Despite making up less than 1% of the normal flora of the gastrointestinal tract it is found in the majority of intra-abdominal abscesses. Other Gram-negative bacilli that can be found in abscesses are of course coliforms (*Escherichia coli*, *Klebsiella*, etc.) or other anaerobic bacteria, such as *Fusobacterium*. However, these are less commonly found than *Bacteroides*. *B. fragilis* causes abscess formation because of the unusual polysaccharide in the cell wall of the organism, which has positively charged NH_2 groups and negatively charged COO groups. The capsular material extracted from *Bacteroides* induces sterile abscess formation if injected into animals.

Most capsular polysaccharides extracted from bacteria are either neutral or have negatively charged groups and do not induce abscess formation. **44**

References

Hofstad T (1992) Virulence factors of anaerobic bacteria. *Eur. J. Clin. Microbiol. Infect. Dis.* **11**, 1044–1048.

Sanders CV & Aldridge KE (1992) Current antimicrobial therapy for anaerobic infections. *Eur. J. Clin. Microbiol. Infect. Dis.* **11**, 999–1011.

45 A serviceman returning from Belize was admitted to hospital. He gave a history of being unwell a week before admission with a fever and headache. These symptoms resolved, but the day before admission he became pyrexial again and on examination was found to be jaundiced and to have an elevated blood urea. Urine was collected and inoculated into a semi-solid agar medium, which after 2 days became turbid and was examined by dark ground microscopy (Fig. 45.1). Serum was also collected for serology.

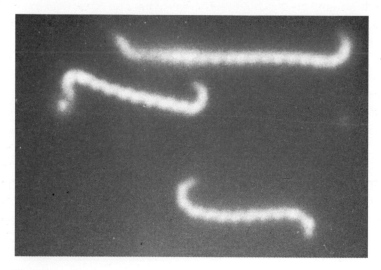

Fig. 45.1

Questions
1 What is your diagnosis?
2 How is the illness transmitted?
3 How should the patient be treated?

1 The patient has a severe form of leptospirosis called Weil's disease, characterized by hepatorenal failure, anaemia and altered consciousness. Typically it is a biphasic illness with a primary phase of pyrexia, myalgia and headaches, which may last for a week. The symptoms improve for a day or two, only to be followed by a recurrence of a temperature accompanied by a variety of other signs and symptoms. The spectrum of the disease can range through a mild feverish illness, without any predominant secondary stage; an aseptic meningitis; to the most severe form of the illness, Weil's disease, with widespread nervous system, renal and hepatic involvement.

   The illness is caused by pathogenic *Leptospira interrogans*, of which there are many serotypes, any of which can cause Weil's disease. Serotypes that are most commonly isolated from patients are *L. autumnalis*, *L. canicola* and *L. icterohaemorrhagiae*, which is particularly found in patients who have been abroad.

   During the first phase of the illness, leptospires can be isolated from the blood, as the symptoms at this stage are caused by a leptospiraemia. Antibodies to *Leptospira* develop during the second week of the illness and *Leptospira* can be isolated from the urine. *Leptospira* can be seen in both the blood and urine by dark ground microscopy, but the organism should be confirmed by culture. Serology is usually performed using the microagglutination test.

2 Animal reservoirs of *Leptospira*, such as rats, dogs or coypu, are the source of human infection. The animals excrete infected urine into water sources and humans become infected from contact with the contaminated water. The *Leptospira* enter the body through skin abrasions or conjunctiva. In the UK, agricultural workers, miners or sewage workers are most at risk of acquiring an infection. Individuals who have aquatic pastimes, for example, white-water canoeists, may also be at risk.

3 The antibiotic treatment for leptospirosis is benzylpenicillin or tetracycline. In patients with Weil's disease additional medical treatments will be required to alleviate the systemic effects of the illness, for example, dialysis for renal failure. Individuals who work in a high-risk environment and sustain an injury, such as miners, should receive tetracycline prophylaxis.

45 Reference

Kuriakose M (1990) Leptospirosis: clinical spectrum and correlations with seven simple laboratory tests for early diagnosis in the Third World. *Trans. R. Soc. Trop. Med. Hyg.* **84**, 19–21.

An elderly patient who had been visiting the New Forest some weeks 46 previously presented to her general practitioner complaining of fatigue, headache and joint pains. On examination the general practitioner noticed a circular erythematous lesion on her ankle; she said this had followed an insect bite. Figure 46.1 shows an insect that may have bitten the patient.

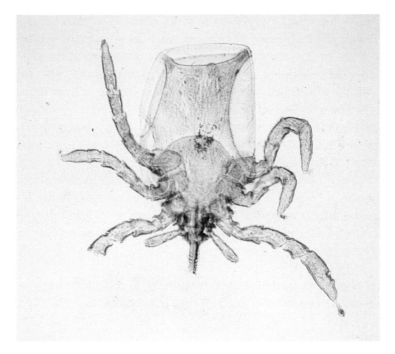

Fig. 46.1

Questions
1 What is the insect and what relevance does it have to her illness?
2 How should she be treated?

46 Answers

1 Figure 46.1 shows a tick. Ticks are vectors for an organism called *Borrelia burghdorferi*, which is the cause of Lyme disease. Rodents and deer may act as reservoirs for the organism. Lyme disease was first recognized as a clinical entity on investigation of an outbreak of an illness, in which arthritis was a prominent feature, in Lyme, Connecticut in the USA. The illness initially presents with a temperature and non-specific systemic symptoms, such as myalgia and headache. There is also a spreading annular erythematous lesion at the site of the tick bite. This is called erythema chronicum migrans. The primary phase of the illness lasts about a month; the signs and symptoms then resolve. This can be followed weeks or months later by evidence of musculoskeletal, cardiac or neurological damage. Chronic arthritis, skin lesions and nerve damage may occur months to years after the initial infection.

Routinely the diagnosis of Lyme disease is serological, although it is possible to isolate *B. burghdorferi* from tissue specimens. Because antibodies may take several weeks to develop, serological diagnosis of early infections is problematical and the diagnosis is principally a clinical one.

2 Lyme disease is treated either by giving a cephalosporin, such as cefotaxime or ceftriaxone, or by giving tetracycline.

References

Aguero-Rosenfeld ME, Nowakowski J, McKenna DF, Carbonaro CA & Wormser GP (1993) Serodiagnosis in early Lyme disease. *J. Clin. Microbiol.* **31**, 3090–3095.

Barbour AG & Fish D (1993) The biology and social phenomena of Lyme disease. *Science* **260**, 1610–1616.

A patient who had AIDS was readmitted to hospital, following treatment for *Pneumocystis* pneumonia, with retinitis caused by cytomegalovirus (CMV). A Hickman line was inserted and the patient was treated with ganciclovir. The patient's previous history included an attack of *Pneumocystis* pneumonia 1 year before his current episode, and Kaposi's sarcoma, for which he had received radiotherapy. His current CD4 count was 50 mm³. During his course of treatment for CMV retinitis, he became pyrexial and anaemic and complained of diarrhoea. Foscarnet was substituted for the ganciclovir but the anaemia persisted. Blood cultures and faeces were sent to the microbiology laboratory, where the organism (Fig. 47.1) was detected in both specimens with a Ziehl–Neelsen stain.

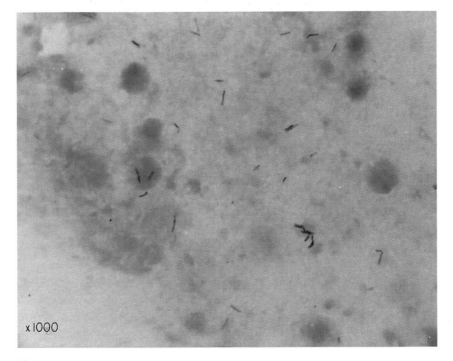

x 1000

Fig. 47.1

Questions
1 What is the likely identity of the organism?
2 How would you manage this patient?

47 Answers

1 The acid-fast microorganism is most likely to be *Mycobacterium avium-intracellulare* (MAI). Disseminated infection with MAI may occur in up to 50% of patients with AIDS. Infection typically occurs late in the course of AIDS, when the patients have often had other opportunistic infections, such as *Pneumocystis* pneumonia. In up to 30% of patients, disseminated infection occurs consecutively with another opportunistic infection, as in this case—CMV retinitis. The CD4 count is usually below $100/\mu l$ when disseminated infection occurs. The patient complains of non-specific symptoms of night sweats, weight loss and fatigue and has a low-grade temperature. Diarrhoea may be a feature and the patient may be anaemic—this is caused by erythrocyte hypoplasia.

MAI is a group of closely related organisms that are ubiquitous in the environment. They are found in soil and water and can be detected in portable water supplies. The organisms are serologically heterogeneous and some serotypes are called *M. avium*, others *M. intracellulare*. *M. avium* is the organism that causes infection in AIDS patients.

2 As this patient is symptomatic he should be treated. MAI is resistant to the standard antituberculous antibiotics, but synergy can be demonstrated if ethambutol and rifampicin are combined. Various regimens have been used to treat symptomatic disseminated infection, for example, ethambutol + rifampicin + amikacin + ciprofloxacin; or ethambutol + rifampicin + clofazimine + amikacin. In some regimens rifabutin has been substituted for rifampicin because it is more active than rifampicin against MAI on *in vitro* testing. In some instances steroids are given to suppress symptoms. Patients from whom MAI has been isolated from a specimen, such as faeces or bronchoalveolar lavage, and who are asymptomatic are usually not treated, although currently controversy exists over the role of rifabutin in primary prophylaxis for disseminated MAI.

References

Ellner JJ, Goldberger MJ & Parenti DM (1991) *Mycobacterium avium* infections and AIDS: a therapeutic dilemma in rapid evolution. *J. Infect. Dis.* **163**, 1326–1335.

Guthertz LS, Damsker B, Bottone EJ, Ford EG, Midura TF & Janda JM (1989) *M. avium* and *M. intracellulare* infections in patients with and without AIDS. *J. Infect. Dis.* **160**, 1037–1041.

Two weeks after returning from a holiday in Malta, a 36-year-old man complained of headaches, night sweats, fatigue and joint pains. He was pyrexial and blood cultures were taken. A Widal test gave a result of O less than 1:40; H160 and an agglutination test for brucellosis was negative at 1:160. Blood cultures were negative after 48 h and the patient's signs and symptoms resolved. Over the following 6 weeks the patient had recurrences of his symptoms, principally headache and fatigue, and additionally complained of backache. On examination he was noted to have hepatosplenomegaly and a liver biopsy revealed granuloma. A repeat Widal test gave a result of O less than 1:40; H160, an agglutination test for *Brucella* was negative at a dilution of 1:160, but one of the original blood cultures taken at the onset of the patient's illness grew the organism shown in Fig. 48.1.

48

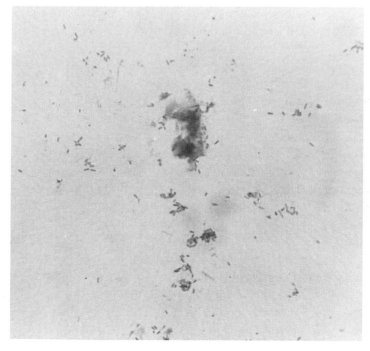

Fig. 48.1

Questions
1 What is your diagnosis?
2 What is your interpretation of the serological results?
3 How would you treat the patient?

48 Answers

1 The photograph shows small Gram-negative bacilli and clinically the patient has brucellosis. There are several species of *Brucella* — *B. melitensis, B. abortis, B. suis* and *B. canis*. The animal reservoirs are sheep and goats; cattle; and pigs and dogs, respectively and they are transmitted to humans through skin abrasions, via the respiratory route or by consuming dairy products made with unpasteurized milk, such as goat's cheese. The incubation period is 2–3 weeks. The acute illness is characterized by fever, headache, night sweats and joint pains. It may also present with an acute confusional state. The symptoms abate but the patient often has recurrences (hence, the name undulant fever). Hepatosplenomegaly develops as the organism becomes sequestered in macrophages and monocytes.

Granulomata are present in both organs. Osteomyelitis, meningoencephalitis or endocarditis may also occur. The chronic illness is also characterized by fatigue and anxiety.

2 In the acute stage an agglutinating immunoglobulin M (IgM) antibody response develops, which may occasionally show a prozone phenomenon. This is caused by blocking antibodies preventing agglutination by the anti-*Brucella* IgM antibodies. If the patient's serum is not sufficiently diluted (thereby diluting out the blocking antibodies), a false-negative result will be obtained. This is why the first serum specimen was negative because the serum has to be diluted to 1:10 000 in order to detect the agglutinating IgM antibodies. In the chronic stage of the illness (the second specimen), agglutinating antibodies are negative but IgG anti-*Brucella* complement-fixing antibodies can be detected.

The Widal test may be used to detect antibodies to *Salmonella typhi* and will be unaffected by an infection with *Brucella*. The high levels of H antigen reflect a previous typhoid vaccination.

3 The optimal treatment for brucellosis is tetracycline and streptomycin. The tetracycline should be given for 2–3 months and the streptomycin for the first month. Alternatively, rifampicin and tetracycline can be used, both given for 3 months.

Co-trimoxazole is equally effective in treating brucellosis, but there is a higher relapse rate than the other antibiotics after treatment has stopped.

References

48

Sanchez Sousa A, Torres C, Campello MG *et al.* (1990) Serological diagnosis of neurobrucellosis. *J. Clin. Pathol.* **43**, 79–81.

Shekabi A, Shakir K, El-Khateeb M *et al.* (1990) Diagnosis and treatment of 106 cases of human brucellosis. *J. Infect.* **20**, 5–10.

Viruses

Abbreviations

Hepatitis B virus

Hepatitis B virus	HBV
Hepatitis B surface antigen	HBsAg
Antibody to hepatitis B surface antigen	Anti-HBs
Antibody to hepatitis B core antigen	Anti-HBc
Antibody to hepatitis B core antigen immunoglobulin M	Anti-HBc IgM
Hepatitis B e antigen	HBeAg
Antibody to hepatitis B e antigen	Anti-HBe

Hepatitis A virus

Hepatitis A virus	HAV
Antibody to hepatitis A virus	Anti-HAV
Antibody to hepatitis A virus immunoglobulin M	Anti-HAV IgM

Hepatitis C virus

Hepatitis C virus	HCV
Antibody to hepatitis C virus	Anti-HCV

A 21-year-old man who gave a history of having multiple male sexual
partners over the past year presented with jaundice. On further questioning he admitted to having pale stools and dark urine. Clinical examination
revealed a slightly enlarged liver with some right hypochondrial tenderness. His liver function tests are shown below—normal range is indicated
in parentheses:

Total bilirubin	360 μmol/l (3–17 μmol/l)
Aspartate transaminase	1100 IU/l (11–55 IU/l)
Alkaline phosphatase	370 IU/l (100–280 IU/l)

A blood sample was sent to the virology laboratory for hepatitis B
serology. The results were as follows:

HBsAg	Positive
HBeAg	Positive
Anti-HBc	Positive
Anti-HBc IgM	Positive

Questions

1 How would you interpret these results?
2 How would you manage this patient?
3 What proportion of recently infected adults become carriers of HBV?
  What is the definition of a HBV carrier?
4 Is this patient likely to become a carrier? Explain your answer.
5 (a) What are the indications for active immunization with HBV
    vaccine?
  (b) Should this individual have been immunized before he developed
  an acute HBV infection?

Answers

1 These results indicate that the patient has an acute HBV infection as he is HBsAg and anti-HBc IgM-positive.

2 Further management and advice to the patient should be as follows.

(a) Management of the patient's acute illness. The treatment of an acute HBV infection is conservative, with most patients being treated on an outpatient basis. However, the patient's liver function, coagulation profile (prothrombin time) and HBV status (HBsAg, HBeAg, anti-HBe and anti-HBs) should be monitored into convalescence. The patient should be advised not to drink alcohol whilst he has an acute hepatitis.

(b) Determination of the possible source of infection. Bearing in mind the routes of transmission of HBV (sexual, perinatal from mother to child and percutaneous), an attempt must be made to identify the source of infection. Of note is that the patient gave a history of having multiple male sexual partners over the preceding year. Other possible routes of transmission, for example, needle-sharing in an injecting drug user, should also be considered.

(c) Management of sexual and close household contacts. The patient's sexual and other close household contacts should be tested for evidence of a current (incubating, acute or carrier state) or past HBV infection. Sexual contacts who have *no* evidence of either should receive a full course of active immunization with hepatitis B vaccine. Passive immunization with hepatitis B immunoglobulin is also recommended for sexual contacts where it is possible to date a recent exposure. It is sensible to give the first dose of HBV vaccine to sexual partners whilst awaiting the serological results—if the sexual partner is subsequently found to be immune to HBV or to have a current HBV infection, immunization can then be discontinued. Susceptible close household contacts should receive a full course of active immunization with HBV vaccine. They do not require passive immunization with hepatitis B immunoglobulin.

(d) The patient should be counselled about the infectivity of his blood and warned of the dangers of sharing razors, toothbrushes and any other potentially blood-contaminated implements. He should also be told not to donate blood and counselled about the use of a condom until he is no longer infectious (i.e. HBsAg-negative).

(e) As it is most likely that the patient acquired his HBV infection sexually, he should be counselled about the acquisition of sexually

transmitted diseases in general and human immunodeficiency virus
(HIV) in particular.

3 A total of 5–10% of newly infected adults will become persistent carriers of HBV. This is defined as the persistence of HBsAg in the patient's serum for more than 6 months after infection.

4 This patient is *unlikely* to become a carrier of HBV. The jaundice associated with an acute HBV infection is thought to be the result of an immune-mediated attack on hepatocytes expressing HBV antigens. Patients who become acutely ill with jaundice are therefore unlikely to become HBV carriers as these clinical symptoms are associated with a brisk immune response. In contrast, individuals with an asymptomatic infection are more likely to progress to a chronic infection. The latter scenario is the norm in perinatally infected infants who seldom develop an acute hepatitis, but in whom chronic carriage develops in the majority of cases.

5 (a) Indications for active immunization with hepatitis B vaccine include the following:
• injecting drug users;
• patients with multiple sexual partners, particularly prostitutes (men and women), homosexual and bisexual men;
• close contacts (household and sexual) of a patient with an acute HBV infection or an HBV carrier;
• babies born to mothers who either are HBV carriers or have had an acute HBV infection during pregnancy;
• patients receiving multiple blood transfusions or blood products, for example, haemophiliacs;
• relatives responsible for the administration of blood products (e.g. to haemophiliacs);
• health care and laboratory workers who have contact with blood or blood-contaminated body fluids;
• patients in chronic renal failure;
• staff and patients in residential accommodation for the mentally handicapped.
(b) Yes, the patient should have received active immunization with HBV vaccine prior to developing an acute infection, as susceptible individuals who have multiple sexual partners (particularly homosexual and bisexual men) are at risk of being infected with HBV.

49 References

Gilson RJC (1992) Sexually transmitted hepatitis: a review. *Genitourin. Med.* **68**, 123–129.

HMSO. Hepatitis B. In: *Immunisation against Infectious Diseases 1992*. HMSO Publications UK, 110–119.

Lau JY & Wright TL (1993) Molecular virology and pathogenesis of hepatitis B. *Lancet* **342**, 1335–1340.

A 24-year-old injecting drug user is noted to be mildly jaundiced when attending his local needle exchange clinic. On further questioning he admitted to feeling generally unwell with mild right hypochondrial pain and anorexia. A blood sample was sent to the virology laboratory for hepatitis serology. The laboratory results obtained were as follows:

Hepatitis A serology
Total anti-HAV   Positive
Anti-HAV IgM   Negative

Hepatitis B serology
HBsAg   Negative
Anti-HBc   Positive
Anti-HBs   Positive
Anti-HBc IgM   Negative

Hepatitis C serology
Anti-HCV not detected

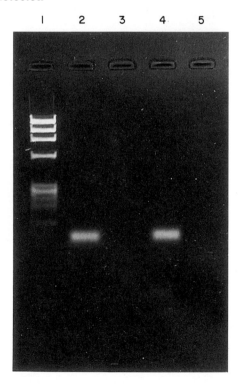

Fig. 50.1

50 Questions

1 How would you interpret these results?

2 Do these results exclude an acute HCV infection? Justify your answer.

3 Examine Fig. 50.1. This is a photograph of an ethidium bromide-stained agarose gel showing the amplification of HCV ribonucleic acid (RNA) using the polymerase chain reaction (PCR). The primers, which amplify a 60 bp segment of the HCV genome, are located in the highly conserved 5' non-coding region.

The photograph shows the following:

Lane 1   Molecular-weight marker

Lane 2   Amplified HCV RNA derived from the patient's serum

Lane 3   HCV-negative control

Lane 4   HCV-positive control

Lane 5   HCV-negative control

(a) What does this demonstrate?

(b) What do you conclude from this?

4 (a) What is the most likely route of infection in this patient?

(b) What are the other possible routes of transmission of this virus?

5 Should you be surprised at the patient's HBV and HAV serological results? Justify your answers.

Answers

50

1 (a) Hepatitis A: these results indicate past infection and immunity to HAV.
(b) Hepatitis B: these results indicate past infection and immunity to HBV.
(c) Hepatitis C: no anti-HCV response was detected.

2 No, anti-HCV seroconversion may be delayed for several months after an acute HCV infection. The currently available serological assays, which are based on a combination of structural and non-structural proteins derived from the HCV genome, are therefore not appropriate for diagnosing an acute HCV infection.

3 (a) Figure 50.1 demonstrates the detection of complementary DNA (cDNA) derived from HCV RNA in the patient's serum by selective amplification using PCR.
(b) The presence of serum HCV RNA in the absence of a HCV-specific antibody response is highly suggestive of an acute HCV infection (except in profoundly immunosuppressed patients, who may have a suboptimal immune response). This is the only currently available method of diagnosing an acute HCV infection.

4 (a) Percutaneous inoculation in an injecting drug user sharing needles.
(b) Other possible routes of transmission include the following avenues.
• Blood transfusion. Prior to the introduction of blood donor screening for anti-HCV, HCV was the major cause of post-transfusion non-A, non-B hepatitis. Blood donors are now screened for anti-HCV in many countries and this has led to a marked reduction in the incidence of post-transfusion HCV infection. However, transmission may still occur by this route, as the currently available serological assays will fail to detect the acutely infected blood donor (see above).
• Needlestick injuries. Other groups at risk of parenteral exposure are health care workers sustaining a needlestick injury from an HCV-infected patient.
• Sexual transmission. There is evidence that HCV can be transmitted sexually, but the efficiency of transmission is low.
• Transmission from mother to child. This has been documented, but the frequency with which this occurs remains to be defined.

5 No, injecting drug users are at risk of acquiring blood-borne viral infections, including HCV, HBV and HIV. Although HBV and HIV are often sexually transmitted, they both may also be acquired by percutaneous inoculation, for example, needle-sharing in injecting drug users, tattooing, acupuncture and chiropody.

There is also an increased risk of HAV infection in injecting drug users. Whilst the injection of infected material is a rare possibility, it is likely that a poor standard of hygiene is a more important cause.

References
Alter HJ, Purcell RH, Shih JW *et al.* (1989) Detection of antibody to hepatitis C virus in prospectively followed transfusion recipients with acute and chronic non-A, non-B hepatitis. *N. Engl. J. Med.* **321**, 1494–1500.

Garson JA & Tedder RS (1993) The detection of hepatitis C infection. *Rev. Med. Virol.* **3**, 75–83.

A 13-week pregnant woman was seen for the first time at a hospital antenatal clinic. As part of her routine antenatal care a blood sample was sent to the virology laboratory for testing for HBsAg. After performing an initial screening test for HBsAg, the laboratory elected to test for the other HBV markers.

51

The completed results were follows:

HBsAg	Positive
HBeAg	Positive
Anti-HBc	Positive
Anti-HBc IgM	Negative

Questions
1 How would you interpret these results?
2 How would you manage:
   (a) this woman's pregnancy?
   (b) this woman's labour and delivery?
   (c) the infant in the postpartum period?
   Justify all of your answers.
3 What further management and advice could you offer the patient and her family?

Answers

1 These results are consistent with a hepatitis B carrier of high infectivity (HBsAg and HBeAg-positive with no detectable anti-HBc IgM).

2. Management should be as follows.

(a) The pregnancy. The pregnancy should be managed as a normal pregnancy, except that invasive prenatal diagnostic techniques should be avoided. Whilst the major route of transmission of HBV from a mother to her infant is perinatally, *in utero* infection may occasionally result from an antepartum haemorrhage with mixing of maternal and fetal blood. Invasive fetal diagnostic techniques, for example, chorionic villus sampling and amniocentesis, may also lead to mixing of maternal and fetal blood. If possible, their use should therefore be avoided in the HBV-infected mother. Alternative non-invasive diagnostic techniques, for example, ultrasound, are preferable.

(b) Labour and the delivery. Fetal monitoring—fetal blood sampling and the use of scalp electrodes should be avoided where possible. The use of an external transducer is preferable.

Staff and infection control—as this woman is a HBV carrier of high infectivity, by definition her blood will be highly infectious. It is therefore important that staff who assist at the delivery are known to be immune to HBV (either naturally or as a result of immunization with HBV vaccine). If an elective Caesarean section is performed, the local hospital infection control guidelines for operation on an HBV-infected patient should be followed. Once again, staff involved in the operation should be immune to HBV. Blood or blood-contaminated body fluid spills should be thoroughly cleaned and disinfected, in accordance with local hospital policy.

(c) HBV prophylaxis in the infant. The infant should be given a combination of active and passive prophylaxis against HBV infection. Passive immunization (in the form of hepatitis B immunoglobulin) together with the first dose of HBV vaccine (active immunization) should be given as soon as possible after birth and certainly within 48h. The hepatitis B immunoglobulin and vaccine should be available within the hospital (by prior arrangement) to facilitate immediate administration. Prophylaxis of the infant is important, as HBV transmission from mother to infant may occur in the perinatal period. The majority of infected infants become HBV carriers (possible because of immunological immaturity). These carriers may then go on to develop chronic hepatitis, cirrhosis and hepatocellular carcinoma.

3 Further management of the patient and her family. This should include the following.

(a) Management of sexual and close household contacts. Sexual and household contacts should be tested for evidence of a current (incubating, acute or carrier state) or past HBV infection. Those with no evidence of either a current or past HBV infection should receive active immunization with HBV vaccine. Sexual partners should also receive passive immunization with hepatitis B immunoglobulin when it is possible to date a recent exposure.

(b) Management of the patient. The patient should be assessed from a hepatological point of view. This includes baseline liver function tests and possibly ultrasound imaging of the liver. Referral to a hepatologist may be required. In general, therapeutic options (not recommended for use in pregnancy) include the use of α-interferon, but the response to such treatment is often poor, with only 30–50% of patients seroconverting from HBeAg to anti-HBe.

(c) General advice. This includes counselling the patient about the infectivity of her blood. She should not share toothbrushes, razors or any other potentially blood-contaminated implements. If her sexual partner is susceptible to HBV infection, the couple should use a condom until immunity has been established.

Reference

HMSO. Hepatitis B (1992) In: *Immunisation against Infectious Diseases*. HMSO Publications UK, 110–119.

52 A 20-year-old woman presented to her general practitioner with jaundice. Of relevance in her history was the fact that she had recently returned from travelling in Africa. She gave a history of feeling generally unwell for several days before becoming jaundiced with fever, malaise, right hypochondrial pain, anorexia and nausea. Her general practitioner sent a blood sample to her local virology laboratory for analysis.

Questions

1 Taking into account the patient's travel history, what is the most likely diagnosis? Justify your answer.
2 The results obtained from the virology laboratory included the following:

Hepatitis A serology

Total anti-HAV	Positive
Anti-HAV IgM	Positive

   How would you interpret these results?
3 How would you manage both the patient and her contacts?
4 Briefly discuss the spectrum of disease associated with infection with this virus.
5 How is this virus transmitted?
6 Could this patient have been offered any form of prophylaxis before travel? If yes, what?

1 An acute HAV infection. HAV is endemic in many tropical and sub-tropical areas. Infection is common where there is overcrowding and poor sanitation. In addition, common source outbreaks may be associated with faecal contamination of drinking water. The patient's history of travel to developing countries in Africa is therefore of importance.

2 The serological profile is that of an acute HAV infection as the patient has detectable serum anti-HAV IgM.

3 Management.
(a) Of the patient. Acute infection with HAV is usually a mild illness. Management is supportive and hospitalization is not necessary in the majority of cases, although occasionally intravenous hydration is indicated for patients with severe nausea and vomiting. The patient should be advised not to drink alcohol whilst she has an acute hepatitis.
(b) Of her contacts. Spread of HAV may be prevented by the use of normal human immunoglobulin for close household contacts. It must be remembered that this may not prevent infection, but only modify the disease course.

4 The spectrum of disease associated with infection with HAV is as follows:
(a) asymptomatic infection;
(b) anicteric hepatitis;
(c) icteric hepatitis;
(d) fulminant hepatitis.
   Children have a higher proportion of subclinical or asymptomatic infections than adults and, when symptomatic, the illness is generally milder and of shorter duration. Prodromal symptoms include malaise, fever, anorexia, nausea, vomiting and right hypochondrial pain. The development of jaundice is usually accompanied by dark urine and pale stools. There is no carrier state of HAV and, in the majority of cases, the illness is benign and self-limiting. However, occasionally a fulminant hepatitis may occur.

5 Transmission of HAV may occur through the following avenues.
(a) The faecal–oral route through close contact between individuals. This is often related to conditions of overcrowding and poor hygiene.

(b) Faecal contamination of food and water. Water-borne outbreaks are associated with faecal contamination of drinking water. Food-borne transmission of HAV may occur as a result of eating raw or partially cooked shellfish which has been cultivated or caught in polluted water. Contamination of food may also occur by food-handlers with an acute HAV infection.

(c) Percutaneous exposure. Percutaneous exposure to blood or serum may infrequently lead to the transmission of HAV. This is a rare occurrence, as the viraemia associated with an acute HAV infection is short-lived and there is no carrier state.

6 Yes, this patient could have been offered prophylaxis against HAV infection prior to travel. Either passive or active immunization could have been used.

(a) Passive immunization. Passive immunization with normal human immunoglobulin may offer short-term protection against HAV. This may be used for people travelling for short periods of time.

(b) Active immunization with HAV vaccine. HAV vaccine is an inactivated vaccine. It is recommended for use in individuals from developed countries who are frequent travellers to HAV-endemic areas or who intend staying for more than 3 months in such areas. This vaccine has been shown to be both safe and immunogenic.

Where possible, individuals should be tested for anti-HAV before the administration of normal human immunoglobulin or HAV vaccine. If they are found to be immune, no prophylaxis is required.

References

HMSO. Hepatitis A (1992) In: *Immunisation against Infectious Disease*. HMSO Publications UK, 104–109.

Tilzey AJ, Palmer SJ, Barrow SJ *et al*. (1992) Clinical trial with inactivated hepatitis A vaccine and recommendations for its use. *Br. Med. J.* **304**, 1272–1276.

A 2-year-old child was admitted to hospital with diarrhoea. She had vomited once, but this was not a prominent feature on presentation. The casualty officer who examined her decided to admit her to the children's ward as she was dehydrated. A stool sample was sent to the virology laboratory to determine the cause of the child's diarrhoea.

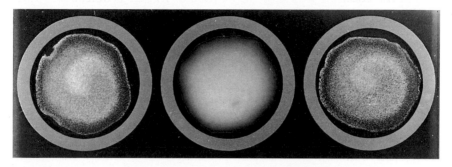

Fig. 53.1 Left, positive control; centre, negative control; right, patient sample.

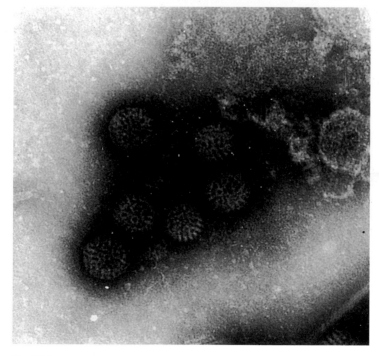

Fig. 53.2

53 Questions

1 What precautions should be taken on admission of this child to the ward?
2 What are the most common viral causes of endemic childhood diarrhoea in the UK?
3 Examine Fig. 53.1. This shows a method of rotavirus detection.
   (a) What test is this? Describe what you see.
   (b) What are the principles of this test?
   (c) Name a shortcoming of this test.
   (d) Name an alternative method of antigen detection.
4 Figure 53.2 shows an electron micrograph prepared from the stool sample taken from the patient.
   (a) What do you see?
   (b) What advantage does this method have over antigen detection systems?
   (c) What do you think are the major limitations of this method of diagnosis?

Answers

1 Local hospital infection control measures should be adhered to. This should entail the isolation of a patient with diarrhoea in a single room to prevent the spread of the causal agent to other patients and staff members in the ward. Basic hygiene, such as hand-washing before and after attending to the patient, is of paramount importance.

2 Rotaviruses, followed by adenoviruses and astroviruses.

3 (a) Figure 53.2 shows a latex agglutination test. Clumping of the latex particles can be seen with the positive control and the patient's stool sample. No clumping is observed with the negative control.
(b) Antibodies directed against rotavirus antigens are fixed to the latex particles. If the stool sample contains rotavirus, agglutination of the latex particles will be observed.
(c) This method targets a specific virus — in this case rotavirus — as antibodies directed against rotavirus antigens are fixed to the solid phase (latex particles). Other viral causes of diarrhoea will not be detected.
(d) An alternative method for rotavirus antigen detection is by enzyme immunoassay.

4 (a) Rotavirus particles.
(b) Electron microscopy allows the virologist to detect, in addition to rotaviruses, other viruses which may also cause diarrhoea. This provides, therefore, a broader 'catch-all' approach.
(c) The virus must have a distinctive morphology, otherwise it will be impossible to recognize. Actual viral particle count is also important. A sufficient number of viral particles must be present to make a certain diagnosis — usually in the region of 10^9 virus particles per gram of faeces.

Reference

Blacklow NR & Greenberg HB (1991) Viral gastroenteritis. *N. Engl. J. Med.* **325**, 252–264.

54 A 7-year-old child was taken to her general practitioner with a rash that was mainly centripetal in distribution, with lesions being most prominent on the abdomen. On examination the child had a temperature of 37.5°C. The skin rash consisted of papules, vesicles and scabs.

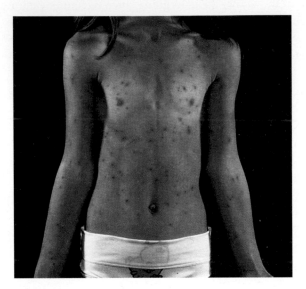

Fig. 54.1

Questions
Examine Fig. 54.1.
1 What is your clinical diagnosis? Justify your answer.
2 How would you confirm the clinical diagnosis in the laboratory?
3 What complications may occur?
4 What group of children is likely to develop severe disease?
5 For how long would you expect the child to be infectious?
6 What therapeutic options are available?

Answers

1 The diagnosis is that of varicella or chickenpox. The clinical presentation of varicella, as described in this child, is that of a rash which is classically centripetal in distribution, appearing on the trunk and the face and then spreading to involve other areas of the body. The skin lesions, which appear as successive crops over a period of 2–4 days, progress from macules and papules to vesicles which then break down with crust formation. Prodromal symptoms may be present for a few days before the onset of the rash.

2 The diagnosis of varicella in the otherwise healthy child is usually a clinical one. However, under certain circumstances, for example, if there is some uncertainty in the clinical diagnosis, laboratory confirmation may be required.

This may be achieved by one of the following techniques.

(a) Demonstration of herpesvirus particles by electron microscopy in material scraped from the base of one of the skin lesions or in aspirated vesicular material. It is not possible to differentiate the various herpesviruses (e.g., herpes simplex virus and varicella-zoster virus) by electron microscopy and so a positive result must be interpreted together with the patient's clinical condition.

(b) Demonstration of the presence of varicella-zoster virus in material taken from the skin lesions by:

• viral culture;

• direct demonstration of varicella-zoster virus antigen using immunofluorescence.

(c) Demonstration of the appropriate specific serological response to varicella-zoster virus. This may be achieved by demonstrating a rise in varicella-zoster virus-specific antibody using an acute and convalescent serum sample or alternatively by the detection of a varicella-zoster virus-specific IgM response.

3 Complications of varicella include the following conditions.

(a) Secondary bacterial infection of the skin lesions. This may increase scarring.

(b) Encephalitis.

(c) Varicella pneumonia.

(d) Haemorrhagic chickenpox.

(e) Reye's syndrome.

54 **4** Varicella (chickenpox) in the immunocompromised patient, child or adult has a significant morbidity and mortality. These patients may develop a progressive disease with involvement of multiple organs, including the lungs and central nervous system.

5 The patient is considered infectious from approximately 48 h before the onset of the rash until all of the vesicles have crusted over and there is no new vesicle formation.

6 In the normal, otherwise healthy child management is usually supportive only. This includes the use of topical antipruritic agents and antibiotics when there is a secondary bacterial infection. Antipyretics (other than aspirin, which is associated with the development of Reye's syndrome) may also be indicated. Practical measures such as cutting fingernails to minimize trauma as a result of scratching are important. The use of the antiviral drug acyclovir in the immunocompetent patient is controversial: some experts consider that its use is only justified when there is evidence of complications, for example, pneumonia. Others consider that, as acyclovir is both safe and effective, as many patients as possible should be treated. All agree that prompt treatment of the immunocompromised child or adult with acyclovir is indicated and many would extend this to include otherwise healthy adults as well.

Reference

Balfour HH & Wood MJ (1992) Acyclovir therapy is indicated for varicella in individuals with normal immunity. *Rev. Med. Virol.* **2**, 3–7.

A 19-year-old college student presented to his general practitioner complaining of malaise, fever and a sore throat. On clinical examination the patient had cervical lymphadenopathy accompanied by a pharyngitis and a faint morbilliform rash. The general practitioner sent a blood sample for haematological and viral analysis.

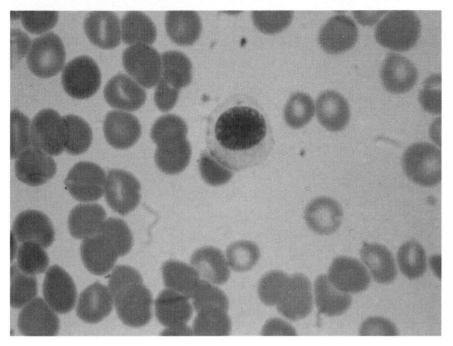

Fig. 55.1

Questions

1 Examine Fig. 55.1. This shows a stained peripheral blood smear. Describe what you see.
2 What is your provisional diagnosis?
3 Based on the clinical information, the following virological investigation was done:

Epstein–Barr virus (EBV) serology

Monospot	Positive
Viral capsid antigen (VCA) IgG	Positive (titre: 1280)
VCA IgM	Positive
Early antigen (EA) IgG	Positive (titre: 160)

What do these results indicate? Justify your answer.

55
4 Outline the principle of the monospot test. What are its shortcomings?

5 Is it always necessary to do full EBV serology in addition to a monospot?

6 What complications may occur?

7 How would you manage this patient?

8 Name three other viruses that can cause a similar syndrome.

1 This illustrates an atypical mononuclear cell.

2 The haematological findings taken together with the clinical presentation of the patient are consistent with the diagnosis of infectious mononucleosis (IM) or glandular fever.

3 These results are consistent with an acute EBV infection. The monospot, which detects heterophile antibody, is positive. Heterophile antibodies are of the IgM subclass and agglutinate red blood cells from species other than humans. They are usually present in an acute EBV infection and remain detectable for 1–6 months. In addition, IgM antibodies to VCA are also present, providing further evidence for the diagnosis of an acute EBV infection in this patient. The presence of detectable levels of EA IgG provides supportive evidence for the diagnosis of an acute EBV infection, but this is less specific, as raised EA IgG levels may be seen in viral infections other than EBV.

4 This is a rapid slide test for the detection of heterophile antibody. The original Paul–Bunnell test involved the incubation of patient serum with sheep erythrocytes. Visible agglutination indicated a positive result. The test was made more specific by a differential absorption step which utilized a guinea-pig kidney suspension to absorb out Forssman-type antibodies and ox erythrocytes to absorb out heterophile antibody. The rapid slide test or monospot is a modification of the original Paul–Bunnell test which uses stabilized horse erythrocytes in the place of sheep erythrocytes. The differential absorption test is as described for the Paul–Bunnell test.

The monospot test has a number of shortcomings.
(a) A false-negative result may occur, particularly in children under 12 years of age.
(b) Patients with chronic IM or postviral fatigue syndrome may occasionally have detectable heterophile antibody.
(c) False-positive results may be found in other medical conditions, for example, in patients with lymphoproliferative disorders.

5 No, it is not always necessary to do full EBV-specific serology. Detectable heterophile antibody (a positive monospot) in a patient with a clinical picture of IM, together with the presence of circulating atypical

55 lymphocytes, is usually sufficient to make the diagnosis in the majority of cases.

6 Complications associated with an acute IM include:
(a) splenic rupture;
(b) neurological complications, including encephalitis and Guillain–Barré syndrome;
(c) tracheal obstruction;
(d) the development of chronic mononucleosis;
(e) haematological complications, including aplastic anaemia and thrombocytopenia.

7 Management of these patients is usually supportive. There is no specific antiviral therapy.

8 A glandular-fever-like illness may occur with:
(a) a primary cytomegalovirus infection;
(b) a primary infection with HIV-1;
(c) an adenovirus infection.

References

Crawford DH & Edwards JMB (1990) Epstein–Barr virus. In: *Principles and Practice of Clinical Virology*, 2nd edn (Zuckerman AJ, Banatvala JE & Pattison JR, eds), 103–128. John Wiley, Chichester.

Hotchin NA & Crawford DA (1991) The diagnosis of Epstein–Barr virus-associated disease. In: *Current Topics in Clinical Virology* (Morgan-Capner P, ed.), 115–140. Laverham Press, Salisbury.

An 8-month-old child was taken to her general practitioner with a history of high fever which lasted for 48 h. On lysis of the fever the infant developed a rose-pink macular rash.

Taking into account the history and clinical presentation of this child, examine Fig. 56.1.

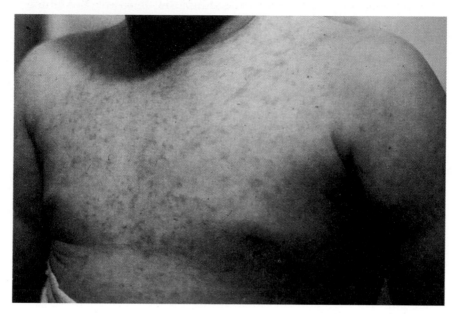

Fig. 56.1

Questions

1 What is the most likely clinical diagnosis?
2 What is the causative agent?
3 How would you confirm the diagnosis?
4 How is this infection acquired?
5 List other possible disease associations of this virus.

56 Answers

1 Roseola infantum or exanthem subitum.

2 Human herpesvirus 6 (HHV-6).

3 In the vast majority of cases the diagnosis of roseola infantum is made clinically. However, the clinical diagnosis may be confirmed serologically by the demonstration of HHV-6-specific IgM. Isolation of HHV-6 is not practical as it requires the patient's peripheral blood mononuclear cells to be cultured in the presence of phytohaemagglutinin and then co-cultured with stimulated lymphocytes.

4 Current knowledge of the epidemiology of HHV-6 infection suggests that HHV-6 is acquired early in life, probably by salivary transmission.

5 It has been suggested that HHV-6 may be associated with the following clinical syndromes:
(a) postviral fatigue syndrome;
(b) hepatitis;
(c) central nervous system disease, including encephalitis and meningitis;
(d) pneumonitis in recipients of bone marrow transplants;
(e) graft rejection in renal transplant recipients;
(f) lymphoproliferative disorders.
     It must be emphasized, however, that the many of the above associations remain to be proven.

References

Fox JD, Briggs M, Ward PA & Tedder RS (1990) Human herpesvirus 6 in salivary glands. *Lancet* **336**, 590–593.

Yamanishi K, Okuno T, Shiraki K *et al*. (1988) Identification of human herpesvirus-6 as a causal agent for exanthem subitum. *Lancet* **i**, 1065–1067.

A child presented with erythema of the cheeks (Fig. 57.1). This was fol- 57
lowed by the development of a lacy reticular rash. Figure 57.2 illustrates
the appearance of this rash. On the left is an adult patient with a laboratory proven parvoviras B19 infection. A lacy reticular rash is visible on her
legs. On the right is an uninfected control (for purposes of comparison).

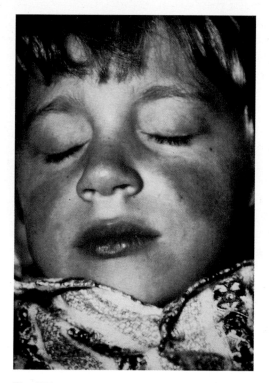

Fig. 57.1

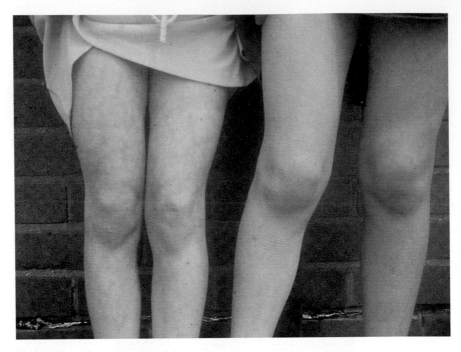

Fig. 57.2

Questions

1 What is the most likely diagnosis?
2 What is the causative agent?
3 Briefly describe the clinical presentation of infection with this virus in a normal, previously healthy child.
4 Describe the pathogenesis of infection with this virus.
5 What are the complications that may be associated with infection with this virus?
6 How would you confirm your clinical diagnosis in this case?
7 How would you manage this patient?

1 Erythema infectiosum (also known as fifth disease).

2 Parvovirus B19.

3 In a typical case of erythema infectiosum, the erythematous phase starts off with a redness of the cheeks with relative circumoral pallor. This is followed by the development of a maculopapular rash. Subsequent central clearing of the involved areas gives the rash a lacy reticular appearance. It is important to realize that, whilst typical cases of erythema infectiosum are easy to recognize clinically, the exanthem associated with B19 infection may vary from a fleeting rash to a florid erythematous exanthem.

4 Infection with B19 is usually acquired via the upper respiratory tract. This is followed by a viraemia with a lytic infection of red blood cell precursors, leading to a drop in haemoglobin with an associated reticulocytopenia. This first phase of the illness, which occurs about 1 week after infection with B19, may be accompanied by non-specific clinical symptoms, for example, pyrexia. The second phase of the illness, that of the rash, occurs about 15–18 days after infection and is thought to be immune-complex-mediated.

5 Complications include the following conditions.
(a) Joint involvement. Arthritis and arthralgia, most often affecting adult females, are the most common complications.
(b) Infection in pregnancy. This may result in fetal loss. Obvious fetal damage in the form of hydrops fetalis may also occur.
(c) An aplastic crisis in patients with chronic haemolytic anaemia, for example, sickle-cell anaemia.
(d) A remitting or relapsing anaemia in the immunocompromised patient, for example, those with congenital immunodeficiencies or AIDS. This is the result of a persistent B19 infection.

6 The diagnosis of the exanthematous phase of infection with B19 is made by demonstrating the presence of B19-specific IgM in the patient's serum.

57　7 Management of the patient is supportive. Analgesia may be required for the joint symptoms.

References

Anderson MJ, Jones SE, Fisher-Hoch SP *et al.* (1983) Human parvovirus: the cause of erythema infectiosum (fifth disease). *Lancet* **i**, 1378.

Public Health Laboratory Service Working Party on 'Fifth' Disease (1990) Prospective study of human parvovirus B19 infection in pregnancy. *Br. Med. J.* **300**, 1166–1170.

A 5-year-old child was taken to his general practitioner with a disseminated maculopapular rash, as shown in Fig. 58.1. According to his mother
the rash first appeared on his head and then spread to involve the rest
of his body. No constitutional symptoms were present. On clinical
examination there was evidence of suboccipital and postauricular
lymphadenopathy. Of relevance was the fact that the child did not receive
combined measles, mumps and rubella (MMR) vaccine in the second year
of life.

58

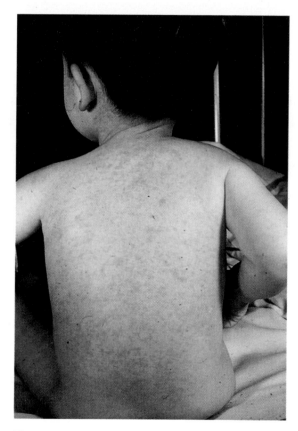

Fig. 58.1

Questions
1 What is the most likely clinical diagnosis? Justify your answer.
2 What is your differential diagnosis?
3 What complications may be associated with infection with this virus?
4 How would you confirm your clinical diagnosis in the laboratory?
5 What risks are associated with infection with this virus in pregnancy?

58 Answers

1 The clinical features are consistent with the diagnosis of rubella. The presence of a maculopapular rash together with suboccipital and postauricular lymphadenopathy are suggestive of rubella. The child has also never been immunized against rubella.

2 A number of viruses may cause a rubelliform rash, for example:
(a) enteroviruses;
(b) parvovirus B19;
(c) alphaviruses, such as chikungunya and Ross river virus, in endemic areas.

3 Complications include the following conditions
(a) Arthritis and arthralgia. Whilst this is uncommon in children and adult males, joint complications frequently occur in postpubertal females.
(b) Thrombocytopenia.
(c) Encephalitis.

4 The diagnosis of rubella is usually made serologically, by demonstrating either a rise in rubella-specific antibody titre or the presence of rubella-specific IgM. In most cases an IgM antibody capture enzyme immunoassay or radioimmunoassay for the detection of rubella-specific IgM is used. Viral culture is not routinely used, as a serological diagnosis is both more reliable and quicker.

5 Rubella infection in pregnancy may result in a congenital infection of the fetus. The risk of an adverse fetal outcome is greatest in the first trimester of pregnancy when infection may result in a spontaneous abortion or the development of the congenital rubella syndrome. This syndrome is a combination of defects which usually includes heart, eye and hearing abnormalities with or without mental retardation and microcephaly. At birth the infant may have hepatosplenomegaly, thrombocytopenia, petechiae, purpura and jaundice. Other features of the syndrome, for example, diabetes, may only become apparent later in life. Maternal rubella after the first trimester of pregnancy may also result in fetal damage, but this is not as severe, as organogenesis is complete, with deafness and retinopathy being the only likely fetal abnormalities.

Reference

Best JM & Banatvala JE (1990) Rubella. In: *Principles and Practice of Clinical Virology*, 2nd edn (Zuckerman AJ, Banatvala JE & Pattison JR, eds), 337–374. John Wiley, Chichester.

59 A child presented with a 2-day history of irritability and fever followed by the development of a bilateral parotid swelling, as shown in Fig. 59.1. Of importance in the history was the fact that the child had not received the combined measles, mumps and rubella (MMR) vaccine in the second year of life.

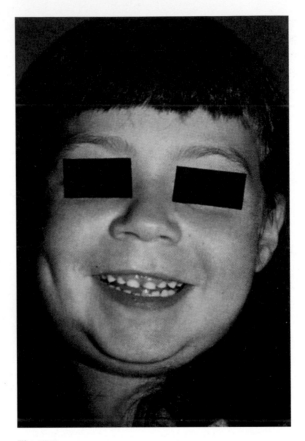

Fig. 59.1

Questions

1 What is your clinical diagnosis?
2 How would you confirm your diagnosis?
3 What are the complications associated with infection with this virus?
4 How would you manage the child?

1 Mumps.

2 The diagnosis may be confirmed either by the demonstration of a mumps-specific antibody response or by the isolation of the mumps virus.
(a) Virus isolation may be attempted from saliva or urine samples.
(b) A serological diagnosis of a mumps infection may be made by demonstrating the presence of mumps-specific IgM or a rise in mumps-specific antibody titre. The latter method of serological diagnosis requires acute (taken at the time of illness) and convalescent (taken 10–14 days later) serum samples to be collected from the patient and tested in parallel to demonstrate the rise in antibody titre.

3 Mumps may be complicated by the following conditions.
(a) Meningitis or encephalitis.
(b) Hearing loss—in most cases this is transient, but it may occasionally be permanent.
(c) Pancreatitis.
(d) Orchitis in males—approximately 20% incidence after puberty.
(e) Oophoritis in females—approximately 5% incidence after puberty.
(f) Arthritis and arthralgia.

4 There is no specific antiviral therapy. Analgesics may be required for pain relief, especially in postpubertal males with orchitis.

Reference

Leinikki P (1990) Mumps. In: *Principles and Practice of Clinical Virology*, 2nd edn (Zuckerman AJ, Banatvala JE & Pattison JR, eds), 375–388. John Wiley, Chichester.

60 A 2-year-old child presented with a history of febrile upper respiratory tract infection. His clinical condition deteriorated, with a worsening cough, dyspnoea and tachypnoea necessitating admission to hospital.

On clinical examination the child had obvious evidence of respiratory distress with rib retraction and an elevated respiratory rate. On auscultation of the chest diffuse wheezing was audible. A chest X-ray showed hyperinflation of both lung fields. A diagnosis of acute bronchiolitis was made and the child was admitted to the paediatric ward. A nasopharyngeal aspirate was collected to be sent to the virology laboratory.

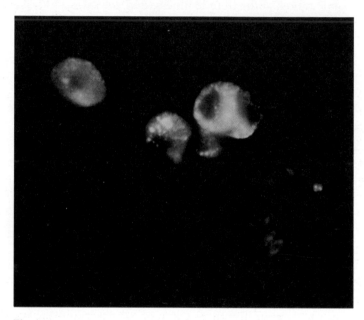

Fig. 60.1

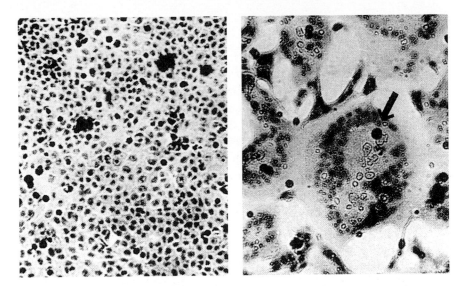

Fig. 60.2 Left, uninoculated cell culture control; right, cell culture inoculated with patient's sample.

Questions

1 What is the most common cause of bronchiolitis?
2 Examine Fig. 60.1. This shows a method of viral antigen detection. The virus sought in this case is the most common cause of bronchiolitis.
  (a) What laboratory test is this?
  (b) What does this demonstrate?
  (c) Outline the principle of this technique.
  (d) What are your therapeutic options? How would you administer this?
  (e) What precautions should be taken on admission to the ward?
3 The nasopharyngeal aspirate was also inoculated into an appropriate cell culture system. This was examined daily and on day 5 certain changes were noted, as shown in Fig. 60.2 (right) (indicated with an arrow). The photographs of the uninoculated cell culture control and the cell culture that has been inoculated with the patient's sample are taken at equal magnification.
  (a) Describe what you see. What does this demonstrate?
  (b) How would you confirm the presence of a specific aetiological agent?
  (c) Why is conventional viral culture a useful additional investigation?

Answers

1 Respiratory syncytial virus (RSV).

2 (a) Immunofluorescent staining of cellular material prepared from the nasopharyngeal aspirate taken from the child.

(b) The presence of RSV antigens in the nasopharyngeal aspirate.

(c) Cellular material contained in the nasopharyngeal aspirate is fixed onto a glass slide. Antibody to RSV, which has been tagged with a fluorescent dye (fluorescein), is left on the cells for approximately 30 min before being washed off. If any RSV antigens are present, the antibody with the fluorescein dye will be bound to the infected cells and the resultant fluorescence can be visualized under an ultraviolet microscope.

(d) An antiviral agent, ribavirin, has been used for treating RSV infections. It is administered via small-particle aerosol. The indications for its use are not well defined but it is generally recommended for RSV infections in premature or immunocompromised infants as well as those with underlying cardiac or pulmonary problems. Most infants, however, simply require supportive care, for example, oxygen therapy and adequate hydration.

(e) RSV is a highly contagious virus. Infants admitted to hospital require immediate isolation, and appropriate infection control measures must be taken to prevent the spread of the virus to staff members (who often only develop a mild upper respiratory tract infection) and other children in the ward. Spread of RSV appears to require close contact with respiratory secretions from an infected individual and probably occurs through large-particle aerosols or fomites. Hand-washing is therefore of critical importance in the prevention of nosocomial transmission of RSV.

3 (a) Clear differences are visible between inoculated and uninoculated cell cultures. In the inoculated cell culture large syncytia are visible. These are indicative of a cytopathic effect due to a syncytia-forming virus, for example, RSV, measles or mumps.

(b) This may be done by immunofluorescence to detect a specific viral antigen (see above).

(c) Although RSV is the most common cause of bronchiolitis, other viruses, for example, parainfluenza viruses, may also occasionally cause bronchiolitis. Viral culture, unlike viral antigen detection which targets a specific virus, allows for the detection of other possible causal agents in a child with bronchiolitis.

60

References

Hall CB (1990) Respiratory syncytial virus. In: *Principles and Practice of Clinical Virology*, 2nd edn (Zuckerman AJ, Banatvala JE & Pattison JR, eds), 253–266. John Wiley, Chichester.

Hall CB, McBride JT, Walsh EE *et al.* (1983) Aerosol ribavirin treatment of infants with respiratory syncytial virus infection. A randomised double-blind study. *N. Engl. J. Med.* **308**, 1443–1447.

61 A 30-year-old man presented to his general practitioner in the winter of 1993 with a history of headache and fever together with a dry cough and quite pronounced muscular aching. His nose was also blocked and his eyes watery.

Questions
1 What is your clinical diagnosis?
2 How would you confirm your clinical diagnosis?
3 What complications are associated with infection with this virus?
4 How would you manage the patient?

1 The clinical features are suggestive of an influenza virus infection. The presence of a fever together with myalgia, headache and upper respiratory tract symptoms is consistent with the clinical diagnosis of influenza.

2 The clinical diagnosis may be confirmed by the following tests.
(a) The detection of influenza virus antigen in respiratory secretions by, for example, immunofluorescence.
(b) Viral culture of respiratory secretions.
(c) The detection of an influenza virus-specific serological response. This is a retrospective diagnosis and is made by demonstrating a rise in specific antibody in the patient's serum. An acute serum sample is taken as soon as possible after the onset of illness and tested in parallel with a convalescent sample taken 14 days later.

3 The following may complicate an infection with influenza virus.
(a) Pneumonia. This may either be a primary viral pneumonia or a secondary bacterial pneumonia, the latter occurring more commonly. *Staphylococcus aureus* is the most frequent cause of a secondary bacterial pneumonia, with *Streptococcus pneumoniae* and *Haemophilus influenzae* occurring less frequently. A primary influenza viral pneumonia is most frequently seen in patients with underlying cardiac disease, although it may also occur in previously healthy individuals.
(b) Other respiratory complications. A tracheobronchitis may occur, particularly in patients with chronic obstructive airways disease, and in the elderly.
(c) Reye's syndrome. Reye's syndrome is an encephalopathy together with fatty degeneration of the liver which has been described in association with a number of viral infections, including influenza A and B, varicella-zoster virus and enteroviruses. The development of this syndrome has been linked to the ingestion of salicylates.
(d) Myositis and myoglobinuria.
(e) Cardiac complications. Influenza has been associated with the development of a myocarditis, but this is a rare complication.
(f) Central nervous system complications. Influenza virus infections have been implicated in the development of Guillain–Barré syndrome and viral encephalitis.
(g) Toxic shock syndrome. A secondary *S. aureus* infection following an

61   influenza virus infection may lead to the development of the toxic shock syndrome.

4 The treatment of uncomplicated influenza is usually symptomatic. Bed rest and adequate oral hydration are important. The use of salicylates should be avoided in children in view of the possible association of the use of this drug together with an influenza virus infection in the development of Reye's syndrome. Specific antiviral agents are not widely used, although the drug amantidine has been shown to reduce the duration of the illness in patients with an influenza A infection. Amantidine does not, however, have specific antiviral activity against influenza B. Antibiotics are used to treat secondary bacterial infections.

Reference

Potter CW (1990) Influenza. In: *Principles and Practice of Clinical Virology*, 2nd edn (Zuckerman AJ, Banatvala JE & Pattison JR, eds), 213–238. John Wiley, Chichester.

A 24-year-old man was admitted to hospital via casualty with a history of a recent onset of dyspnoea on exertion and bouts of palpitations. Ten days previously he had suffered a mild influenza-like illness with muscle aches which left him feeling tired. Signs of heart failure were present on examination and electrocardiogram (ECG) changes suggestive of a myocarditis were noted. The cardiac team discussed the case with the clinical virologist and the following samples were sent to the virology laboratory for examination – clotted blood and stool.

62

An extract prepared from the stool sample was inoculated into an *in vitro* cell culture system. On day 7 a viral cytopathic effect suggestive of an enteroviral infection was observed. Supernatant fluid from the cell culture was used to determine the type of enterovirus present in the patient's stool sample.

Examine Fig. 62.1. This illustrates one method of determining the type of enterovirus present.

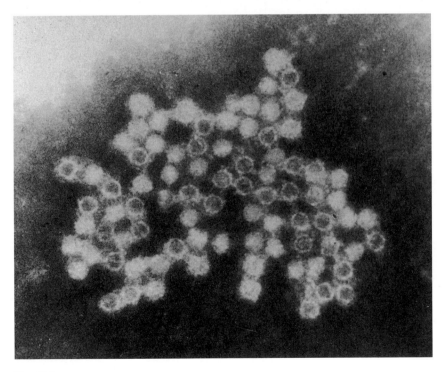

Fig. 62.1

Questions

1 (a) What is this technique called?
   (b) What are the principles of this test?
   (c) What is the clinical significance of the demonstration of enterovirus in a stool sample taken from a patient with a suspected viral myocarditis?

2 Which enteroviruses have been associated with the development of a viral myocarditis?

3 In addition to attempting viral culture, indirect serological evidence may be sought for a recent enteroviral infection. The results were as follows:

Enteroviral serology
Enteroviral-specific IgM: positive

   (a) What do these results indicate?
   (b) What are the clinical significance and limitations of this test result?

4 Unfortunately, the patient died of uncontrolled ventricular dysrythmias. The clinical team requested an autopsy. Postmortem examination of myocardial tissue showed evidence of a myocarditis (damage to the myocardial tissue with an infiltrate of inflammatory cells). How could you confirm the diagnosis of an enteroviral-associated myocarditis using cardiac tissue obtained at postmortem?

1 (a) Immune electron microscopy.

(b) Cell culture supernatant fluid, obtained from the cell culture in which the stool extract was cultured, has been incubated with specific enteroviral antiserum (in this case a pool of Coxsackie B virus antisera) prior to performing electron microscopy. The antiserum links the viral particles together and this results in clumping of virus.

(c) This result demonstrates the presence of a current enteroviral infection in this patient. However, enteroviruses may be shed in both nasopharyngeal secretions and faeces in a proportion of healthy individuals (particularly children). The demonstration of a current enteroviral infection is not therefore necessarily indicative of an enteroviral-associated myocarditis.

2 Coxsackie B viruses are the most common cause of a viral myocarditis. However, other enteroviruses, such as Coxsackie A viruses and echoviruses, have also been associated with the development of a viral myocarditis.

3 (a) These results are consistent with a recent enteroviral infection.

(b) The detection of enterovirus-specific IgM in the patient's serum provides serological evidence of a recent enteroviral infection and therefore raises the possibility of an enteroviral-associated myocarditis. However, as an enterovirus-specific IgM response may persist for 1–6 months after an acute infection, a positive result must be interpreted with some caution as it may be unrelated to the patient's current illness. Serological methods are also frequently unable to determine the type of enterovirus infection.

4 Confirmation of an enteroviral-associated myocarditis may be done by the following techniques.

(a) Viral culture of the myocardial tissue. However, the isolation of an enterovirus from the myocardial tissue is rarely possible.

(b) Detection of enteroviral RNA by nucleic acid hybridization or selective amplification of viral genome using polymerase chain reaction (PCR).

Reference

Muir P (1993) Enteroviruses and heart disease. *Br. J. Biomed. Sci.* **50**, 258–271.

63 A 62-year-old woman was brought into the accident and emergency department of her local hospital after, according to her family, she had had a generalized seizure with subsequent loss of consciousness. Her family had also noted that she had been behaving oddly and complaining of headaches for several days. On clinical examination the patient was comatose with no obvious focal neurological signs. No papilloedema was observed on fundoscopy.

The following special investigations were performed:

Computed tomography (CT) scan
This showed low-density lesions in the temporal lobe region.

Lumbar puncture
After excluding the presence of raised intracranial pressure a lumbar puncture was done.

Analysis of the cerebrospinal fluid (CSF) showed the following
White cell count   40 cells/mm³ with a lymphocyte pleocytosis
Red blood cell count   300 cells/mm³
Protein   0.78 g/l (normal range: 0.15–0.45 g/l)

Electroencephalogram (EEG)
EEG showed slow δ-rhythms and periodic discharges.

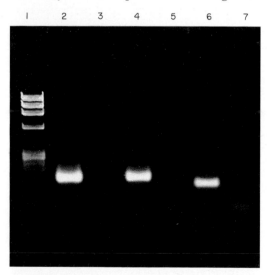

Fig. 63.1

1 What is your provisional diagnosis? Justify your answer.
2 What is your differential diagnosis?
3 Examine Fig. 63.1. This is a photograph of an ethidium bromide-stained agarose gel which illustrates one laboratory method to confirm the diagnosis of this condition:

Lane 1   Molecular-weight marker

Lane 2   Amplification of viral DNA in the patient's CSF sample using herpes simplex virus (HSV-1) primers

Lane 3   Amplification of viral DNA in the patient's CSF sample using HSV-2 primers

Lane 4   HSV-1-positive control

Lane 5   HSV-1-negative control

Lane 6   HSV-2-positive control

Lane 7   HSV-2-negative control

(a) Explain and interpret what you see. What are the advantages and disadvantages of this technique?

(b) How else could the clinical diagnosis be confirmed? What is the disadvantage of this?

4 Describe two further tests that may be used to diagnose this condition. What are the disadvantages of these?
5 How would you treat this patient? Why is rapid treatment essential?

63 Answers

1 Herpes simplex encephalitis (HSE).

The clinical presentation is often as described in this patient. The onset of disease is frequently insidious. The prodromal phase, consisting of non-specific symptoms and signs, such as headache, personality changes, fever and malaise, may persist for 4–10 days. This is usually followed by an abrupt development of more severe central nervous system involvement, for example, a seizure, coma, disorientation or stupor. The CT scan may provide important diagnostic information, but this is not always the case. Low-density lesions in the temporal region of the brain are suggestive of the diagnosis of HSE. The CSF typically shows a mild lymphocyte pleocytosis and the protein may be elevated. The EEG may also provide diagnostically useful information, characteristically showing slow δ-rhythms and periodic discharges. Therefore, the special investigations, taken together with this patient's clinical picture, are suggestive of the diagnosis of HSE.

2 It is of paramount importance to attempt to differentiate HSE from other medical conditions as this will influence the management of the patient. Included in the differential diagnosis are:
  (a) brain abscess;
  (b) tuberculoma;
  (c) cerebrovascular accident;
  (d) tumour.

3 (a) This shows the detection of HSV DNA in the CSF sample taken from the patient using selective amplification of HSV DNA by the polymerase chain reaction (PCR). The amplified HSV DNA is then subjected to agarose gel electrophoresis with subsequent ethidium bromide staining of the gel.

  Amplified HSV-1 DNA derived from the patient's CSF sample can be seen in lane 2. The detection of HSV DNA in the CSF sample obtained from the patient provides laboratory confirmation of the diagnosis of HSE.

  'Nested' PCR, using primers located in the glycoprotein D gene of HSV-1 and the glycoprotein G gene of HSV-2, has been shown to be both a sensitive and specific method of diagnosing HSE. It has the advantage of being less invasive than brain biopsy. However, false-negative results do occasionally occur so, as with all diagnostic techniques, it is important to interpret the result in the context of the

206

patient's clinical condition. In addition, the detection of HSV DNA by PCR is not a routine diagnostic test and is often only available from specialist centres.

(b) The clinical diagnosis of HSE may also be confirmed by the analysis of brain tissue obtained by brain biopsy or at postmortem (histopathologically and by the detection of HSV antigens in or culture of HSV from brain tissue).

A major disadvantage of this method of diagnosis is that brain biopsy is an invasive procedure and is sometimes not a viable option in patient management.

4 The demonstration of intrathecal HSV antibody synthesis and the demonstration of HSV antigens in the CSF.

(a) The measurement of HSV antibody in the CSF requires the parallel measurement of the blood−brain barrier function to exclude the possibility that increased CSF HSV antibody levels may be the result of blood–CSF barrier damage. In addition, intrathecal antibody synthesis may only be reliably detected from 7–10 days after the onset of the neurological symptoms. This limits its usefulness as an acute-phase diagnostic tool.

(b) Tests for HSV antigens in the CSF have been found to be neither sensitive nor specific in the diagnosis of HSE.

5 If a diagnosis of HSE is suspected, the patient should be put on intravenous acyclovir without delay. HSE is a clinical emergency and treatment must not be delayed until laboratory confirmation of the diagnosis is obtained. A delay in treatment may influence both morbidity and mortality.

References

Aurelius E (1993) Herpes simplex encephalitis. Early diagnosis and treatment and immune activation in the acute stage and during long term follow-up. *Scand. J. Infect. Dis.* **89** (Suppl.), 5–62.

Aurelius E, Johannson B, Skoldenberg B & Forsgren M (1993) Encephalitis in immunocompetent patients due to herpes simplex virus type 1 or 2 as determined by type-specific polymerase chain reaction and antibody assays of cerebrospinal fluid. *J. Med. Virol.* **39**, 179–186.

64 A 4-year-old child was taken to her general practitioner by her parents with a 1-day history of fever and irritability. On examination the general practitioner found the child to have neck stiffness. He referred the child to the accident and emergency department at the local hospital. On admission there the child did not appear critically ill, but was clearly irritable and had a temperature of 37.5°C. The casualty officer confirmed the presence of neck stiffness. The remainder of the clinical examination revealed no abnormalities. In particular there were no focal neurological signs.

A lumbar puncture was performed.

Analysis of the cerebrospinal fluid (CSF) showed the following:
White blood cells   100/mm³ with a lymphocyte predominance
Protein   0.68 g/l (normal range: 0.15–0.45 g/l)

Gram staining and bacterial culture of the CSF were both negative.

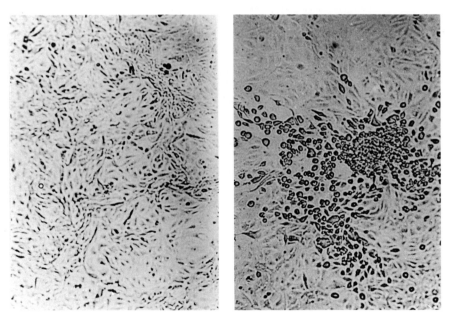

Fig. 64.1 Left, uninoculated cell culture control; right, cell culture inoculated with patient's sample.

1 Why is it important to do bacterial culture and Gram staining of the CSF?
2 A sample of CSF was also sent to the virology laboratory for viral culture. This was inoculated into a monolayer of cells.

 Examine Fig. 64.1. This shows a cell culture monolayer that has been inoculated with the patient's CSF sample. An uninoculated control is included for comparative purposes.
 (a) Explain what you see.
 (b) What is this called?
3 What is the most likely causative agent?
4 How would you confirm your diagnosis?
5 What other viruses may cause meningitis?
6 How would you manage this patient?
7 Would you expect the patient to have residual neurological sequelae following her acute illness?

Answers

1 Although the clinical features and analysis of the CSF are consistent with the diagnosis of an acute viral meningitis, it is important to exclude a bacterial meningitis as this will influence subsequent management of the patient.

2 (a) Rounded dead or dying cells are seen in the cell culture monolayer that has been inoculated with the patient's CSF sample (compare this to the uninoculated control).
(b) This is known as a viral cytopathic effect.

3 An enterovirus.

4 There are a number of enteroviruses that may cause viral meningitis, including coxsackieviruses of both groups A and B, echoviruses and enterovirus 71. In order to provide a more precise diagnosis, the type of enterovirus isolated in cell culture may be further identified using serological tests, for example, neutralization. As the name implies, this entails neutralization of the viral cytopathic effect in cell culture using specific antisera. Cultured virus from the patient's CSF sample is allowed to react with specific antibody before inoculation in cell culture. Because of the number of different types of enteroviruses, pools containing a number of selected antisera are used in the first instance, with further analysis after the identification of a neutralizing pool of antisera. The identification of a neutralizing antiserum then permits identification of the causative virus.

An alternative method of identification is the use of immune electron microscopy, where clumping of the enteroviral particles by a specific antiserum may be observed.

5 Mumps, herpes simplex virus (HSV)-2 and varicella-zoster virus may also cause meningitis.

6 Management is supportive. There is no specific antiviral therapy available.

7 Recovery is usually complete, with no residual neurological sequelae.

Reference 64

McGee ZA & Baringer JR (1990) Acute meningitis. In: *Principles and Practice of Infectious Disease*, 3rd edn (Mandell GL, Douglas RG & Bennett JE, eds), 741–755. Churchill Livingstone, New York.

65 Immunocompromised patients may be unable to deal with viral infections in a normal manner. An immunocompromised state may result not only from the immunosuppressive therapy used after organ transplantation, but also from congenital and acquired diseases or the cytotoxic therapy used to treat many malignancies.

A 31-year-old female underwent allogeneic bone marrow transplantation for acute myeloid leukaemia. In the second month posttransplant she developed a non-productive cough and breathlessness. Her chest X-ray showed a diffuse interstitial pneumonitis.

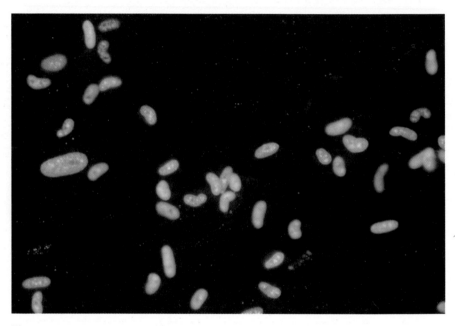

Fig. 65.1

1 What is the most likely viral cause for the patient's pneumonitis?
2 (a) How would you attempt to make a more specific virological diagnosis?
   (b) What laboratory tests could you use?
3 A bronchoalveolar lavage was performed on the patient and a sample was sent to the virology laboratory to investigate a possible viral cause for the patient's pneumonitis.
   Examine Fig. 65.1. This illustrates a rapid method of diagnosing a cytomegalovirus pneumonitis in an immunocompromised patient.
   (a) What is this test called?
   (b) Outline the principles of this test.
   (c) What is the advantage of this method of diagnosis compared to conventional viral culture?
4 How would you treat this patient? Explain the rationale for this therapeutic approach.
5 What other viruses can cause pneumonitis in the immunocompromised patient?

Answers

1 Cytomegalovirus (CMV).

2 (a) A more specific diagnosis may be made by the following techniques.
   • Identification of the causal agent in the affected organ. In an immunocompromised patient an attempt should be made to identify the causative agent at the involved site, in this case the lung. This may be done by demonstrating CMV in bronchoalveolar lavage fluid or lung tissue.
   • Identification of a current CMV infection in the patient. Target organ samples are not always available for analysis and so a presumptive diagnosis may sometimes be made in a patient who has clinical and radiological evidence of a CMV pneumonitis, together with evidence of peripheral shedding of CMV (e.g., in the urine or pharyngeal secretions).
   (b) The following laboratory tests are used.
   • Conventional viral culture.
   • Modified rapid culture or detection of early antigen fluorescent foci (DEAFF).
   • Direct immunofluorescence for viral antigens.
   • Cytology and histopathology. Here, 'owl's eye' inclusions may be seen. Confirmation with a virus-specific test is preferable.
   • Detection of CMV DNA.

3 (a) This modified rapid culture technique is known as the DEAFF test.
   (b) Human fibroblast cell monolayers are inoculated with the clinical sample (in this case, a bronchoalveolar lavage) and examined after 24–48 h using fluorescein-labelled antibodies directed against intermediate–early or early CMV proteins. Fluorescence is then visualized using ultraviolet microscopy.
   (c) DEAFF testing has the advantage of being rapid when compared to conventional viral culture, which may take 2–3 or more weeks before a cytopathic effect becomes evident. A rapid result is essential for the management of the acutely ill patient.

4 A combination of a specific antiviral drug, usually ganciclovir, and intravenous immunoglobulin should be used. CMV pneumonitis in transplant recipients is thought to be immunologically mediated and is associated with the development of graft-versus-host disease. This

understanding of the pathogenesis of CMV pneumonitis in the transplant recipient has led to the development of a rational therapeutic approach. A combination of antiviral and immunotherapy is used. The intravenous immunoglobulin is thought to block the targets of cell-mediated immunity on infected lung cells and ganciclovir limits the viral replication.

5 Other viral causes of an interstitial pneumonitis include:
  (a) adenovirus;
  (b) respiratory syncytial virus (RSV);
  (c) influenza virus;
  (d) parainfluenza viruses;
  (e) herpes simplex virus (HSV);
  (f) varicella-zoster virus.

66

Four months after her bone marrow transplant the patient discussed in case 65 developed the lesions illustrated in Fig. 66.1.

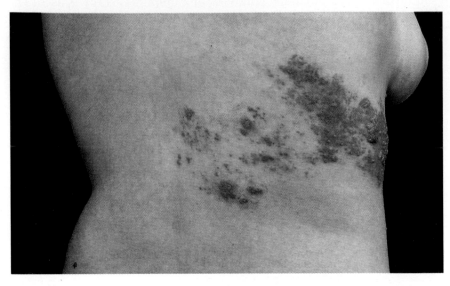

Fig. 66.1

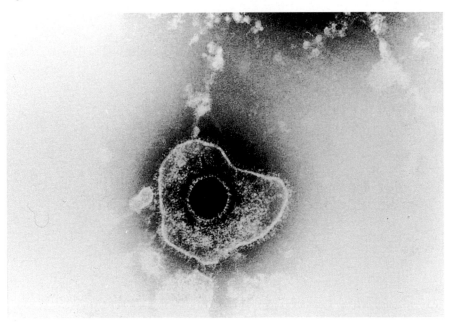

Fig. 66.2

Questions

1 What is this clinical condition?
2 What is the causative agent?
3 (a) How would you confirm your diagnosis in the laboratory?
  (b) One method of diagnosis is illustrated in Fig. 66.2. Describe what you see.
  (c) How would the sample used in this method have been taken from the patient?
  (d) What is the major limitation of this method of diagnosis?
4 How would you treat this patient?

66 Answers

1 Herpes zoster or shingles.

2 Varicella-zoster virus (VZV).

3 (a) The diagnosis of shingles is usually a clinical one. If laboratory confirmation is required, the following may be done.
• Demonstration of the presence of herpesvirus particles by electron microscopy.
• Demonstration of the presence of VZV by viral culture or viral antigen detection.
• Demonstration of a rise in VZV-specific antibody using an acute and convalescent serum sample taken from the patient. As the antibody titre may rise rapidly, the acute sample should be taken as soon as possible after the appearance of the lesions.
(b) This electron micrograph illustrates the presence of a typical herpesvirus particle.
(c) A fresh vesicle is opened with a scalpel and the base of the lesion gently scraped. Alternatively, vesicular fluid may be aspirated from a lesion. The material is placed on a glass slide and sent to the virology laboratory.
(d) The herpesvirus particles of VZV cannot be differentiated from other herpesviruses, for example, herpes simplex virus (HSV), by conventional electron microscopy.

4 This patient should receive specific antiviral therapy, usually acyclovir.

References

Frank I & Friedman HM (1988) Progress in the treatment of cytomegalovirus pneumonia. *Ann. Intern. Med.* **109**, 777–782.

Webster A & Griffiths PD (1991) Treatment of cytomegalovirus infections. In Morgan-Capner P, ed.: *Current Topics in Clinical Virology*, 165–179. Laverham Press, Salisbury.

A 24-year-old man, who had initially been diagnosed as being HIV-positive 8 years before, presented with a right-sided weakness and visual disturbance. His partner had noted a decline in the patient's mental status over the preceding month. Examination confirmed the presence of a right-sided weakness together with a homonymous hemianopia.

The following investigations were done:

CD4 T-lymphocyte count   60/mm³ (normal range: 350–2200/mm³)

Computed tomography (CT) of the brain   Multiple lesions in the white matter with no mass effect

Magnetic resonance imaging (MRI) of the brain   Multifocal lesions involving the white matter consistent with the diagnosis of progressive multifocal leucoencephalopathy (PML)

Cerebrospinal fluid (CSF)   No cells
Protein 0.48 g/l (normal range: 0.15–0.45 g/l)

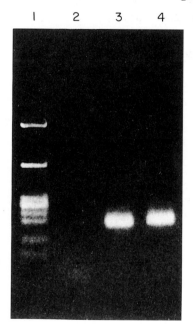

Fig. 67.1

Questions

1 What is PML?
2 What virus is the cause of PML in the overwhelming majority of cases?
3 What is the natural history of infection with this virus?
4 Briefly describe the pathogenesis and clinical features of PML.
5 How can the diagnosis of PML be made?

Figure 67.1 of an ethidium bromide-stained agarose gel illustrates one method of diagnosis, which uses a CSF sample obtained from the patient. Specific viral DNA (the virus that causes PML) has been targeted for selective DNA amplification using the polymerase chain reaction (PCR).

Figure 67.1 shows the following:

Lane 1   Molecular-weight marker
Lane 2   Negative control
Lane 3   Positive control
Lane 4   Amplified viral DNA derived from the patient's CSF

1 PML is a progressive demyelinating disease occurring in individuals with an impaired ceel-mediated immune response.

2 JC virus (JCV).

3 Serological surveys have shown that JCV has a worldwide distribution, with infections in humans usually occurring early in life. The majority of adults have evidence of infection by adulthood. Little is known about the transmission of JCV, but this probably occurs via the respiratory or oral route. After the primary infection the virus establishes a renal and possibly CNS latency. Reactivation of the latent infection may occur during pregnancy and in elderly and immunocompromised patients.

4 PML usually occurs in patients with disordered immunity. It is most likely the result of reactivation of latent virus with subsequent replication in and destruction of oligodendrocytes with loss of myelin. Whether the virus reaches the brain during the primary infection or reactivation is unclear.

   The clinical features of PML obviously depend on the location of the lesions within the central nervous system. However, a visual defect, hemiplegia and alteration of the patient's mental state are common initial manifestations. Seizures may occur but these are rare. Death usually occurs in less than 6 months.

5 The diagnosis of PML may be made through one of the following techniques.
   (a) Radiological imaging. Both MRI and CT are useful in making the diagnosis. Abnormalities in the white matter are seen which have no mass effect or enhancement.
   (b) Examination of the CSF.
   • General analysis. A mild lymphocyte pleocytosis and mildly elevated protein may be seen in the minority of cases.
   • Detection of JCV DNA. More recently, CSF has been used to detect the presence of JCV DNA in patients with suspected PML. JCV DNA may be detected in the CSF of about 80% of patients with PML. This method of diagnosis, which has the advantage of being less invasive than brain biopsy, is illustrated in Fig. 67.1.
   • Demonstration of intrathecal antibody synthesis. A further possible method of diagnosis of PML is the demonstration of intrathecal

synthesis of JCV-specific antibody in the CSF. However, the currently available serological assays are relatively insensitive.

(c) Examination of brain tissue obtained at biopsy or autopsy. The pathological features seen in brain tissue consist of abnormal oligodendroglial cells and bizarre astrocytes. Confirmation of the presence of JCV may be done by electron microscopy, detection of viral antigens or the detection of JCV DNA.

Reference

Major EO, Amemiya K, Tornatore CS, Houff SA & Berger JR (1992) Pathogenesis and molecular biology of progressive multifocal leucoencephalopathy—the JC virus-induced demyelinating disease of the human brain. *Clin. Microbiol. Rev.* **5**, 49–73.

A 25-year-old homosexual man attended the genitourinary medicine clinic at his local hospital for a general health check. He gave a history of having had unprotected anal intercourse with several partners over the last 3 years. No abnormalities were noted on clinical examination. The attending health care worker counselled the client about sexually transmitted diseases, including viral infections. In particular, the possibility of being tested for evidence of HIV infection was discussed. This included a discussion on the meaning and possible consequences of a positive HIV test result.

Questions

1 What viral infections may be transmitted sexually?
2 The patient agreed to have HIV antibody testing. His HIV serology results were as follows:

Screening test

Immunometric enzyme-linked immunosorbent assay (ELISA) for anti-HIV-1 and 2	Positive

Confirmatory tests

Competitive ELISA for anti-HIV-1	Positive
Particle agglutination for anti-HIV-1	Positive

  (a) Why is a combination of serological assays used?
  (b) Outline the principles of each of the above tests.
3 Taking the results of the laboratory tests into account, what is your diagnosis?
4 What further action should be taken regarding this patient's immediate management?

68 Answers

1 The viruses listed below may be transmitted sexually.
   (a) Herpes simplex virus (HSV).
   (b) Human papillomavirus.
   (c) Molluscum contagiosum.
   (d) HIV.
   (e) Human T-cell lymphotropic virus 1 (HTLV-1).
   (f) HBV.
   (g) HCV (transmitted sexually with a low-grade efficiency).
   (h) Cytomegalovirus (CMV).
   (i) Epstein–Barr virus (EBV).

2 (a) Most laboratories within the UK use a combination of various assay types. The screening test used should detect both anti-HIV-1 and anti-HIV-2 (although HIV-2 is rare outside West Africa). It is of paramount importance that the initial serological reactivity is confirmed by a second and perhaps a third test utilizing a different methodology to confirm the specificity of the initial reaction. Sera that give strongly concordant results are considered to be anti-HIV-positive. Discordant or weak reactions should be further investigated using alternative methodology, for example, further antibody testing by Western blotting or HIV antigen or genome detection.

(b) In the immunometric (or 'sandwich') ELISA, HIV antigens are fixed to either a bead or a well (the solid phase) which is then incubated with the patient's serum. Binding of specific antibody (in the patient's serum) is detected by the addition of a second labelled viral antigen.

In the competitive anti-HIV-1 assay the solid phase contains HIV-1-specific antigens. The patient's serum is incubated together with a labelled HIV-1-specific antibody and competitive binding occurs. The resultant colour intensity in the ELISA is therefore inversely proportional to the HIV-1-specific antibody concentration in the patient's serum. In addition to confirming the initial serological reactivity, the competitive anti-HIV-1 ELISA also allows speciation of HIV-1 and HIV-2.

The particle agglutination test consists of gelatin particles coated with HIV-1 antigens which are incubated with the patient's serum. Visible agglutination of the particles is indicative of a positive test result.

3 This patient has serological evidence of a HIV-1 infection.

4 (a) Confirmation of the test result. A second sample should be taken from the patient to confirm the initial diagnosis. This is of paramount importance in view of the serious nature of the diagnosis. Although stringent checks are made within the laboratory and clinic, the very small potential for an error to occur still exists.

(b) Post-test counselling of the patient. A positive HIV test result may be extremely traumatic for the patient. Psychological and emotional support may be required both from the hospital or clinic and within the community.

(c) Medical treatment. In order to have a realistic discussion with the patient about his prognosis, treatment and life expectancy, it is important to establish whether he has an asymptomatic HIV infection or AIDS. This is usually determined on the basis of clinical findings, the timing of the primary infection (seroconversion illness), if known, and repeated CD4 T-lymphocyte counts. When appropriate, the patient should be offered information on suitable prophylactic and treatment regimes and clinical trial participation. He should also be advised to see either a clinic physician or his general practitioner on a regular basis to monitor his clinical condition, CD4 T-lymphocyte counts and any treatment.

(d) Practical advice. The patient should be told about potential infectivity of his blood and body fluids. He should be encouraged (as for hepatitis B) not to share toothbrushes, razors or any implement that could be contaminated with his blood or blood-contaminated body fluids. Counselling should also be given on safer sexual practices. The patient should be advised to tell his general practitioner, dentist and sexual partner(s) of his diagnosis. Sexual partner(s) should be encouraged to come in for counselling and testing.

Reference

Mortimer PP (1993) The virus and the tests. In: *The ABC of AIDS*, 3rd edn (Adler M, ed.). BMJ Publishing Group, London.

69

A 22-year-old man presented to his general practitioner complaining of fever, lethargy, malaise and a sore throat. On clinical examination he had evidence of generalized lymphadenopathy together with a maculopapular rash. The rash was most prominent on the patient's face and trunk.

Questions

1 What is the differential diagnosis of a glandular-fever-like illness?
2 On further questioning the patient gave a history of having unprotected anal intercourse with a number of men over the preceding few months, one of whom was subsequently found to be HIV antibody-positive. He was referred to his local hospital for further investigation. After some discussion with the patient it was decided to investigate him, with his consent, for a possible HIV infection. The opinion of the virologist was sought and the following samples were sent to the laboratory for analysis—clotted blood for HIV antibody and HIV-1 p24 antigen testing and anticoagulated blood for HIV-1 genome detection.

The results obtained were as follows:

HIV antibody testing
Immunometric assay for anti-HIV-1 and 2	Negative
Competitive assay for anti-HIV-1	Negative
Particle agglutination for anti-HIV-1	Negative

HIV antigen testing
HIV-1 p24 antigen	Positive

HIV genome detection
HIV-1 proviral DNA	Detected by selective DNA amplification (polymerase chain reaction—PCR)

What is your diagnosis? Justify your answer.

3 What other clinical features (besides those seen in this patient) may be present?
4 What further virological investigations should be done?
5 How would you treat this patient?

Answers 69

1 A glandular-fever-like illness may be caused by the following conditions:

(a) Viral infections:
- Epstein–Barr virus (EBV);
- cytomegalovirus (CMV);
- adenovirus;
- a primary or acute HIV infection (the seroconversion illness).

(b) Other infections:
- toxoplasmosis.

(c) Other medical conditions:
- leukaemia or lymphoma.

2 The diagnosis is that of a primary or acute HIV-1 infection.

A primary or acute HIV infection (acute seroconversion illness) is included in the differential diagnosis of a glandular-fever-like illness. This occurs 2–12 weeks (usually 2–6 weeks) after infection. It is estimated that at least 50% of the new cases of HIV infection will develop symptoms and signs at the time of the primary HIV infection. These include fever, pharyngitis and lymphadenopathy, together with a maculopapular rash. The clinical presentation in this patient is therefore consistent with an acute or primary HIV infection. Of importance in this patient is his history of having unprotected anal intercourse with a partner who was subsequently found to be HIV-infected. This obviously puts the patient at risk of becoming infected with HIV.

The laboratory results obtained on this patient are also consistent with an acute or primary HIV infection as, at this stage of the infection, HIV-specific antibody may be undetectable. The presence of HIV-1 p24 antigen and HIV-1 proviral DNA in the absence of an HIV-specific antibody response is therefore diagnostic of an acute or primary HIV-1 infection.

3 Other features of a primary HIV-1 infection include diarrhoea, nausea and vomiting, oral candidiasis, ulceration of the oropharynx and anogenital area, headaches, hepatosplenomegaly and a leucopenia. Rarely, meningitis, encephalopathy and neuropathy may occur.

4 Further samples should be obtained from the patient to monitor the development of HIV-specific antibodies.

5 Treatment of a patient with an illness associated with a primary HIV infection is usually supportive. Zidovudine has been used in some cases, but its use in this clinical setting has not yet been established.

References

Niu MT & Schittman SM (1993) Primary human immunodeficiency virus type 1 infection: review of pathogenesis and early treatment in human and animal retrovirus infections. *J. Infect. Dis.* **168**, 1490–1501.

Tindall B & Cooper DA (1991) Primary HIV infection: host responses and intervention strategies. *AIDS* **5**, 1–14.

A 24-year-old woman presented with genital ulceration (Fig. 70.1). This was accompanied by malaise and a low-grade fever. The patient complained of considerable local discomfort with a burning sensation of the external genitalia which preceded the development of the genital ulceration. On questioning she gave no history of previous episodes of genital ulceration. An associated inguinal lymphadenopathy was noted on clinical examination.

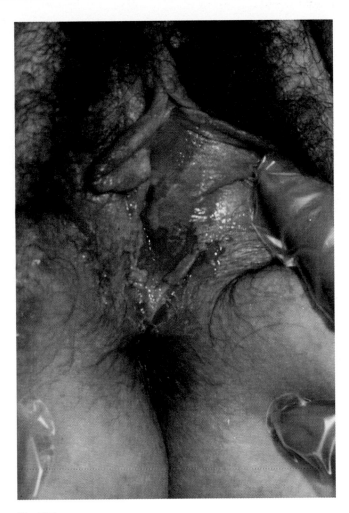

Fig. 70.1

70 Questions

1 What is your clinical diagnosis? Justify your answer.
2 How is this virus transmitted?
3 What complications may be associated with this clinical condition?
4 How would you confirm your clinical diagnosis in the laboratory?
5 What is your differential diagnosis?
6 How would you manage this patient?

1 A primary or initial herpes simplex virus (HSV) infection.

A primary HSV infection occurs when a previously HSV antibody-negative individual acquires their first HSV infection. In contrast, an initial HSV infection describes the first episode of infection at a particular anatomical site. As this patient's HSV antibody status is unknown, she may have either a primary or initial genital HSV infection, both of which occur in a patient with no prior history suggestive of genital herpes. Although an initial infection is usually less severe than a primary infection, both may result in genital ulceration, together with constitutional symptoms such as fever and malaise. In contrast to this, the symptoms associated with recurrent genital HSV infections are generally milder and are usually not associated with constitutional symptoms.

2 HSV (both types 1 and 2) is transmitted through contact with infected lesions or secretions when there is a breach in the integrity of the skin or mucosa. In the case of a primary genital HSV infection, this usually occurs through sexual contact.

3 A primary genital HSV infection may be complicated by:
(a) bacterial superinfection of cutaneous or mucosal lesions;
(b) neurological complications, for example, a radiculitis, urinary retention, neuralgia and meningoencephalitis;
(c) the subsequent development of recurrent genital HSV infections.

4 Laboratory confirmation of the clinical diagnosis is usually done by:
(a) viral culture;
(b) viral antigen detection by enzyme immunoassay or immunofluorescence;
(c) cytology—this may be used to detect cellular changes suggestive of an HSV infection but is of low sensitivity.

5 Genital HSV infection must be differentiated from other causes of genital ulceration, for example:
(a) lymphogranuloma venereum;
(b) chancroid;
(c) syphilis (both a primary chancre and condylomata lata);
(d) granuloma inguinale;
(e) Behçet's syndrome;

70   (f) contact dermatitis;
(g) candidiasis.

6 Initial genital HSV infections are usualy treated with acyclovir. Intravenous acyclovir is the most effective form of treatment but, as this requires hospitalization, this is reserved for patients with very severe disease. Oral acyclovir is used in the majority of cases. Acyclovir has a favourable influence on the disease course, with a reduction in pain and length of time to complete healing. Further management of the patient is largely supportive and includes the use of analgesia, if required, and counselling the patient about the natural history of a genital HSV infection.

References

Stanberry LR (1993) Genital and neonatal herpes simplex virus infections: epidemiology, pathogenesis and prospects for control. *Rev. Med. Virol.* **3**, 37–46.
Whitely RJ & Gnann JW (1992) Acyclovir: a decade later. *N. Engl. J. Med.* **327**, 782–789.

Parasites

A 27-year-old agricultural worker was seen in the outpatient department 4 months after returning from an overland trekking holiday in Africa. He complained of passing blood in his urine and had noticed blood in his semen. There were no associated urinary tract symptoms. Whilst in Africa he had had a febrile illness which resolved without treatment, and he had swum in inland waters.

On examination he was afebrile and well. Rectal examination revealed a nodular prostate but no other abnormalities. Dipstick testing of his urine confirmed haematuria. An eosinophilia of $1.2 \times 10^9/l$ was noted in the blood film. Microscopy of terminal urine (Fig. 71.1) and stool was performed and blood was drawn for serology.

71

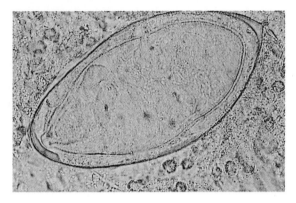

Fig. 71.1

Questions
1 What is the object in Fig. 71.1?
2 What was the likely nature of the febrile illness, and how was it acquired?
3 How else may the diagnosis be made?
4 What are the long-term consequences of infection?
5 What is the treatment of choice?

71   Answers

1 This is an egg of the blood fluke *Schistosoma haematobium*. The adults of this species usually live in the pelvic veins and their eggs migrate through the bladder wall to escape in the urine. If the eggs reach fresh water they hatch to release miracidia which infect water snails. They are distinguished from other schistosome eggs by the terminal spine.

2 It was probably Katayama fever, a form of acute schistosomiasis. As well as fever, patients may have an itchy rash, hepatomegaly and eosinophilia. Infection is acquired from contact with fresh water infested with schistosome-bearing snails. These release infectious cercaria into the water which penetrate the skin and enter the blood stream where they develop into adult flukes.

3 Eggs may also be detected in stools or rectal snips. They may also be found in histological specimens from other sites such as liver, bladder and vulva. The presence of terminal haematuria or haematospermia in a patient with a history of exposure should suggest schistosomiasis. Indirect diagnosis by serology may be helpful, although this does not differentiate between acute, chronic or treated cases.

4 *Schistosoma* eggs elicit a granulomatous reaction in the tissues. This results in scarring and fibrosis of affected organs. Local complications include loss of bladder volume, hydroureter and obstructive renal failure. Some cases may progress to bladder carcinoma. Ectopic eggs in the central nervous system may cause fits and spastic paralysis. Schistosomes may harbour *Salmonella typhi* and be a cause of persistent carriage of this organism after an episode of typhoid fever.

5 Praziquantel. It is well tolerated and effective.

Reference

Cook GC (1990) *Parasitic Disease in Clinical Practice*, 121–140. Springer-Verlag, London.

A 40-year-old female English entomologist presented 1 week after return- **72** ing from a 3-week visit to Mexico. Apart from a mild diarrhoeal illness during the second week of her visit, she had been well. However, a week after her return she developed a fever of 40°C, rigors and some ill-defined upper abdominal pain. In hospital she was found to have epigastric tenderness. Her white blood cell count was elevated, at $13 \times 10^9/l$ (86% neutrophils) and her erythrocyte sedimentation rate was raised at 72mm/h. Later, she developed right shoulder tip pain. A computed tomography (CT) scan of the liver revealed a 10×6cm cavity in the right lobe (Fig. 72.1). This was aspirated, yielding a brownish red odourless opaque fluid. On microscopy the fluid contained moderate numbers of red and white blood cells but no bacteria. Bacterial cultures were negative. The clinical diagnosis was confirmed with a further test.

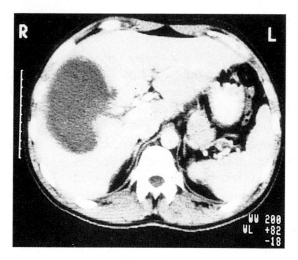

Fig. 72.1

Questions
1 Give the most likely diagnosis and two differential diagnoses.
2 Is it surprising that the causative organism was not seen in the aspirate?
3 How was the diagnosis confirmed?
4 How would you manage the patient?
5 What other disorders can this parasite produce?

72 Answers

1 Amoebic liver abscess (ALA) would best account for her history and signs. Other diagnoses to consider would be a bacterial pyogenic abscess, a necrotic tumour or an infected hydatid cyst. Ultrasonography is a readily available alternative to CT scanning to detect a liver abscess.

2 No. The amoebic trophozoites are only found feeding at the edges of the abscess and are rarely seen in the aspirate.

3 The diagnosis is usually confirmed serologically. Immunofluorescent antibody tests (IFAT) are positive in over 90% of cases of ALA. The cellulose acetate precipitin (CAP) test is usually only positive in active amoebic infection. Other serological tests are also used for this purpose. The detection of amoebic cysts in faeces is of limited use in diagnosing ALA. They are often absent in confirmed cases of ALA and may be present in people with non-amoebic liver abscesses.

4 Aspiration of ALA is usually only necessary if it is large or there is diagnostic confusion. The mainstay of treatment is metronidazole or tinidazole. This should be followed by a course of diloxanide furoate to clear the intestine of cysts. Family contacts of the patient should also be screened for infection and treated if they are found to be carriers.

5 Most cases of *Entamoeba histolytica* infection are asymptomatic. Gut infection ranges in severity from a mild self-limiting diarrhoeal illness through amoebic dysentery to a life-threatening fulminant colitis with mucosal destruction and perforation. Amoebiasis can be confused with ulcerative colitis or Crohn's disease. It is essential to avoid this confusion because corticosteroids which may be given for inflammatory bowel disease may prove fatal in amoebic infections. Amoebic colitis is diagnosed by finding haematophagous trophozoites of *E. histolytica* in fresh warm faecal samples (the so-called hot stool) or in rectal scrapes and biopsies. Serology may be negative in invasive gut infection.

As well as gut and liver infection, *E. histolytica* may cause pulmonary or pleural collections. These are usually due to extension of ALA across the diaphragm. Cutaneous infection, usually seen in the tropics, may occur perianally, where a collection has drained or, rarely, as an isolated necrotic patch of skin.

Reference

Reed SL (1992) Amebiasis: an update. *Clin. Infect. Dis.* **14**, 385–393.

73 A 48-year-old mechanic was seen with a history of abdominal pains, weight loss and malaise. He was born in Trinidad but had lived for many years in the UK. Examination was unremarkable, but a barium meal and endoscopy revealed abnormal duodenal mucosa. Biopsies of small bowel had the features seen in Fig. 73.1. A full blood count showed a mild eosinophilia (eosinophils $0.7 \times 10^9/l$), and on stool microscopy the organisms shown in Fig. 73.2 were seen.

The patient was treated appropriately with repeated courses of albendazole and later ivermectin, but his condition recurred after each course. The results of a further blood test explained his failure to overcome this infection.

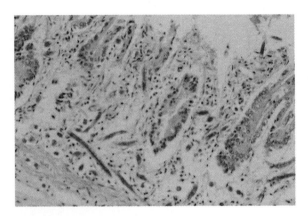

Fig. 73.1

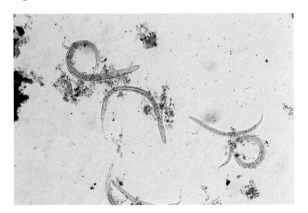

Fig. 73.2

Questions

1 What are the histological features of the biopsy seen in Fig. 73.1 and what are the organisms seen in Fig. 73.2?
2 When did the patient contract the infection?
3 What are the complications of this infection?
4 What did the further blood test show?

Answers

1 Nematode larvae are seen in section in the lumen, epithelium and lamina propria.

   The organisms in Fig. 73.2 are rhabditiform larvae of *Strongyloides stercoralis*. This non-infectious stage may mature to the infectious filariform stage in the intestine or in the environment. Intestinal maturation results in an autoinfective life cycle in which filariform larvae reinvade the body, enter the blood stream, pass via the lungs into the small bowel and develop into adult worms. Environmental maturation results in filariform larvae which pass through the skin to enter the blood stream, or in sexual stages which multiply in warm soil to increase the number of infectious larvae in the environment.

2 He probably contracted the infection in Trinidad. Transmission is rare in temperate climates. The infection is able to persist for very long periods because of the autoinfective cycle described above.

3 The complications of strongyloidiasis include intestinal malabsorption, diarrhoea, pulmonary eosinophilia, asthma, hyperinfection and secondary bacterial septicaemia. This last is thought to occur when large numbers of filariform larvae coated with intestinal flora invade the blood stream.

4 The blood test was positive for antihuman T-cell lymphotropic virus type 1 (HTLV-1) antibodies. This retroviral infection is prevalent in the Caribbean and is associated with hyperinfection and persistent strongyloidiasis. Other predisposing causes of hyperinfection are immunosuppressive disorders, including transplantation and AIDS, and steroid therapy. In patients with a history of probable exposure, *Strongyloides* infection should be excluded before starting immunosuppressive or steroid therapy.

Reference

Cook GC (1990) *Parasitic Disease in Clinical Practice*, 91–101. Springer-Verlag, London.

A 17-year-old Welsh schoolboy was referred to his local hospital for **74** investigation of abdominal pain. He gave a 2-month history of stabbing pains in the right upper abdomen. He lived in a rural sheep-farming area and had a pet dog. On examination he was found to have a tender liver which extended 6 cm below the right costal margin. Liver function tests were normal but there were increased numbers of eosinophils (1.2 × 10^9/l) in the blood film. Abdominal computed tomography (CT) revealed a large cyst in the right lobe of the liver (Fig. 74.1).

Despite appropriate treatment with albendazole the patient was readmitted to hospital as an emergency, with hypotension, tachycardia and severe abdominal pain. The cyst was surgically evacuated. The cyst fluid contained the microscopic structures seen in Fig. 74.2. He made a good postoperative recovery and received two further 1-month blocks of albendazole therapy. One year later, his symptoms had resolved and his liver returned to normal size.

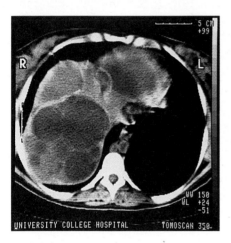

Fig. 74.1

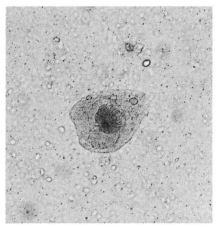

Fig. 74.2

Questions

1 What is the lesion seen on CT scanning?
2 What is the object seen in Fig. 74.2?
3 How is this infection contracted?
4 What complication did the patient develop?
5 How is the diagnosis usually made?

74 Answers

1 It is a hydatid cyst. These are usually single and thick-walled and may contain smaller daughter cysts. These are the tissue stage of the dog tapeworm, *Echinococcus granulosus*, which occurs naturally in sheep. They are most commonly seen in the liver but may occur in other tissues such as spleen, lung and bone. Many cases are asymptomatic and are detected as incidental findings during investigation of other conditions.

2 This is a hydatid protoscolex. The inverted scolex can be seen within, bearing hooks. Protoscolices are produced by the germinal epithelium which lines the cyst. In nature the definitive host (a dog) would consume cysts in sheep offal and the protoscolices would develop in its small bowel to form tapeworms.

3 Hydatid disease is contracted by the inadvertent ingestion of *Echinococcus* eggs. Control is by preventing dogs from consuming un-cooked offal and regular deworming of dogs.

4 The patient suffered a ruptured cyst. This may occur spontaneously or following trauma. It is dangerous because the patients develop high levels of anti-hydatid immunoglobulin E (IgE). When the cyst ruptures, the antigen released may result in anaphylactic shock. Other complications arise when the cyst acts as a space-occupying lesion (e.g. in the brain) or is locally invasive (e.g. in bone).

5 The clinical and radiological features of hydatid disease may suggest the diagnosis. Aspiration is contraindicated as it may release enough antigen to precipitate anaphylaxis or lead to seeding of daughter cysts. In a typical case serology is often used to confirm the diagnosis. Its drawbacks are that it may be negative in long-standing infections and that it cross-reacts with other cestode infections, particularly cysticercosis.

Reference

Horton RJ (1989) Chemotherapy of *Echinococcus* infection in man with albendazole. *Trans. R. Soc. Trop. Med. Hyg.* **83**, 97–102.

A 63-year-old retired man called his general practitioner because of a fever and rigors. He had a past history of chronic bronchitis and had returned from a holiday in the Gambia a month earlier. Whilst there he had taken weekly chloroquine prophylaxis, but had omitted to take it after his return. His doctor diagnosed influenza. Five days later, he collapsed and died soon after admission to hospital. Histological specimens of liver (Fig. 75.1) and spleen taken postmortem showed extensive pigment deposition. Blood samples taken immediately before death were also reviewed (Fig. 75.2).

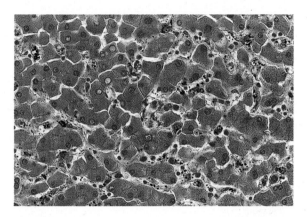

Fig. 75.1

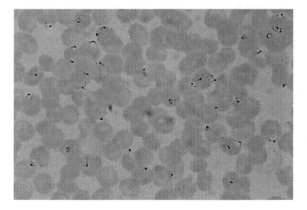

Fig. 75.2

75 Questions

1 What is the diagnosis and are the clinical features of this case unusual?
2 Comment on the antimalarial prophylaxis.
3 How common is this disease in the UK?
4 Why is the diagnosis often missed?

1 This was a fatal case of malaria. This pattern of disease is only seen with *Plasmodium falciparum* infections. The clinical features of this case are not unusual. Malaria can present with diarrhoea and vomiting, headache, joint pain, influenza-like illness, jaundice, cough, fits or shock and sudden death. There is a great potential for misdiagnosis if blood films are not examined. In any febrile patient returning from an endemic area malaria must be considered and excluded as a matter of urgency.

2 Chloroquine alone was not adequate prophylaxis. Chloroquine resistance is now common in *P. falciparum* in many parts of the world, including West Africa. This patient did not take a full course; he should have continued to take prophylaxis for 4 weeks after his return. Protection is not absolute with any antimalarial prophylaxis and travellers should be aware of this fact. It follows that a history of prophylaxis, no matter how obsessively taken, does not exclude a diagnosis of malaria. Advice should also concentrate on avoidance of mosquito bites using bed nets, insect repellents, long sleeves and insecticide sprays.

3 In 1993 the Public Health Laboratory Service Malaria Reference Laboratory recorded 1922 cases of malaria in the UK. Of these, 1060 were due to *P. falciparum*. Five of these patients died.

4 The diagnosis may be missed because of an atypical presentation. Often, it is not even considered because a travel history is not taken: (a) because of a misplaced faith in prophylaxis; (b) because blood films are not taken or are falsely reported as negative; and (c) occasionally because the malaria is contracted in unusual circumstances. Examples of the latter would be transmission by blood transfusion, organ transplantation, needle-sharing amongst intravenous drug users or from the bite of imported malarious mosquitoes, so-called airport malaria. The most common reason is that the diagnosis is not considered.

Reference

World Health Organization Division of Control of Infectious Diseases (1990) Severe and complicated malaria. *Trans. R. Soc. Trop. Med. Hyg.* **84** (Suppl. 2), 1–65.

76 A 35-year-old Maltese man, resident in the UK for 1 year, was reviewed in a specialist AIDS unit with fever, weight loss, malaise and splenomegaly. He had been seropositive for HIV infection for 7 years without major complications. He also had oral candidiasis and axillary and inguinal lymphadenopathy. Blood cultures were negative for mycobacteria and conventional bacteria, but a bone marrow smear showed the organisms seen in Fig. 76.1.

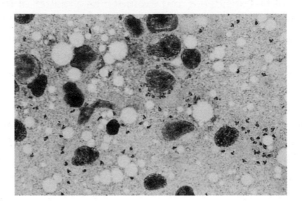

Fig. 76.1

Questions

1 What are the organisms seen in Fig. 76.1 and what is the diagnosis?
2 How is this infection contracted?
3 How may it be treated?
4 What other forms may infection with this parasite take?

Answers

1 They are amastigotes of *Leishmania* species. These are the human stage of this parasite. They are intracellular parasites which multiply in macrophages. In smears the macrophages may rupture and release the parasites. *Leishmania* species may be recognized by the presence of two dark staining bodies of nuclear material. There is a large rounded nucleus and a smaller kinetoplast.

   This patient has infection of the spleen and bone marrow. He has visceral leishmaniasis. In the western Mediterranean this is predominantly an infection of children and is caused by *L. infantum*, which has a reservoir of infection amongst dogs. Recently, cases have been reported in AIDS, where it probably represents reactivation of a dormant infection.

2 Leishmaniasis is transmitted by sandfly bites. These are small blood-sucking insects which may feed on a variety of animals, including humans. Whilst feeding on a *Leishmania*-infected host they ingest amastigotes; these develop into infectious promastigotes which multiply in the sandfly gut and infect the next host on which the fly feeds.

3 Conventional treatment of visceral leishmaniasis is with pentavalent antimony compounds such as sodium stibogluconate. Alternatives include paromomycin and the antifungal drug amphotericin B. In AIDS, relapse is common after therapy.

4 Cutaneous leishmaniasis is the commonest Old-World form. It usually presents as an indolent ulcerating lesion at the site of a bite. Diagnosis is by finding the parasite either in biopsy samples or in slit-skin smears. In the Americas infection may result in a more destructive disease—mucocutaneous leishmaniasis. This results in destructive lesions of the nose and lips, as well as skin lesions.

Reference

Pearson RD & de Queiroz Sousa A (1990) Leishmania species: visceral (kala-azar), cutaneous and mucosal leishmaniasis. In: *Principles and Practice of Infectious Diseases*, 3rd edn (Mandell GL, Douglas RG & Bennett JE, eds), 2066–2077. Churchill Livingstone, New York.

77 A 19-year-old veterinary nurse was seen in outpatients with a 2-week history of malaise, fever and lumps in the neck. Her temperature was 37.4°C and there were multiple cervical, axillary and inguinal lymph nodes. Her throat was normal and her spleen was impalpable. A full blood count was normal and the monospot test was negative. An axillary lymph node was biopsied for diagnostic purposes. The histological appearances are shown in Fig. 77.1.

Fig. 77.1

Questions
1 What is the diagnosis and what is the differential diagnosis for this syndrome?
2 How is the diagnosis usually made?
3 How is the infection contracted?
4 What other syndromes are caused by this parasite?

1 This is acute glandular toxoplasmosis. The lymph node architecture is normal but there is follicular hyperplasia. There are scattered collections of epithelioid cells with pale cytoplasm, forming granulomata. The parasites themselves are rarely seen in biopsy specimens. This protozoal infection is common and often asymptomatic. In this patient it resembles glandular fever. The differential diagnosis would include infectious mononucleosis (IM), primary cytomegalovirus (CMV) infection, HIV infection and lymphoreticular disorders such as lymphoma.

2 The diagnosis is usually made serologically. Rising titres of anti-*Toxoplasma* immunoglobulin G (IgG) measured by latex agglutination is the usual method in a routine laboratory. This can be confirmed in a reference laboratory by the *Toxoplasma* dye test and by the demonstration of anti-*Toxoplasma* IgM antibodies using enzyme-linked immunosorbent assay (ELISA) tests.

3 The life cycle of *T. gondii* is complex. The definitive host is the cat, in which the infection is primarily intestinal. Oocysts are produced in the cat's small bowel and are passed with the faeces into the environment. There, they develop into mature oocysts containing infectious sporozoites. If the oocysts are consumed by a cat the enteric cycle is repeated. If the oocysts are ingested by a non-feline the sporozoites invade the blood stream and settle in the tissues where they multiply and then lie dormant as bradyzoites. The tissue stages are infectious to cats if ingested, resulting in intestinal infection; and to humans, resulting in tissue infection. Human infection is therefore either contracted from an environment contaminated with cat faeces or by the consumption of uncooked meat containing the tissue stages.

4 These are a number of other clinical manifestations of toxoplasmosis.
(a) Congenital toxoplasmosis. If a woman contracts toxoplasmosis during pregnancy, the parasites in her blood can cross the placenta and infect the fetus. This may lead to fetal loss or the congenital *Toxoplasma* syndrome of hydrocephalus, intracerebral calcification and choroidoretinitis.
(b) Ocular toxoplasmosis. Fetal infection acquired in late pregnancy may not be apparent at birth, but may be noticed in childhood or even adult life as a progressive scarring choroidoretinitis.

77 (c) Cerebral toxoplasmosis. The maintenance of *Toxoplasma* bradyzoites in their resting state seems to depend on the integrity of the immune system. In immunosuppressed patients, particularly those with AIDS, this suppressive function is lost and the parasites start to multiply. This occurs particularly in the brain, where focal infections act as space-occupying lesions. They are seen on computed tomography (CT) scan as ring-enhancing structures.

Reference

Joss A & Ho-Yen D (1992) *Human Toxoplasmosis*. Oxford Medical Publications, Oxford.

A 40-year-old office worker was referred from her local hospital with a 2-year history of an itchy rash over her shoulders and waist. More recently, she had developed a swelling in her right axilla. She gave a history of working in rural Cameroon 4 years earlier. On examination she had a rash of small papules over the shoulders, with thickening of the overlying skin and signs of recent excoriation. The axillary swelling was a fleshy lymph node of 2×3 cm. A blood sample showed a raised eosinophil count of $3.3 \times 10^9/l$. Filarial serology was strongly positive. There were no microfilariae in the blood or skin snips, but a test dose of diethyl-carbamazine citrate (DEC) produced a florid papular erythematous reaction in the affected skin (Fig. 78.1) and conjunctival swelling. After a few days she was given ivermectin, which resulted in a marked abatement of her symptoms.

78

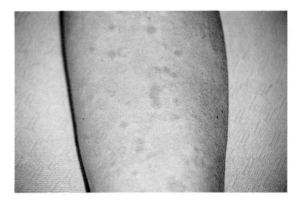

Fig. 78.1 Skin of forearm.

Questions

1 What is the diagnosis?
2 What are the possible long-term consequences of this infection?
3 How is the disease controlled in endemic areas?
4 What is the purpose of the test dose of DEC?

1 Onchocerciasis. This filarial infection is endemic in West and Central Africa and in parts of Central and South America. It is transmitted by blackflies of the genus *Simulium*. These blood-feeding flies have aquatic larvae which live in rapids attached to weed and rocks. Transmission is most intense in the proximity of rapidly flowing water. Infected flies bite exposed areas, injecting infectious microfilariae as they do so. The larvae invade the subcutaneous tissue and develop into adult worms which live in groups in skin nodules. The microfilariae produced by the adult worms live in the skin, which induces a brisk local immune response with migration of eosinophils. This may be responsible for the itching and loss of skin elasticity characteristic of this infection. With scratching, the skin becomes thickened and pigmented, particularly over the buttocks and shoulders.

The clinical diagnosis is usually confirmed by taking superficial skin snips from shoulders, buttocks and thighs. The snips are incubated in saline for a few hours. Any microfilariae present migrate into the saline where they can be identified microscopically. Microfilariae may also be seen in the eyes on slit-lamp examination. The adult worms are seen in histological sections of skin nodules.

2 The main effects of chronic infection are cutaneous and ocular. The thickening of the skin may become very marked and the loss of elasticity may result in premature ageing and 'hanging groin', where enlarged inguinal lymph nodes lose their supporting tissues and become pendulous. The intense itching is a cause of great distress.

More serious is the eye disease due to onchocerciasis. This affects all compartments of the eye causing keratitis, anterior uveitis, choroidoretinitis and optic neuritis. All of these separately, or in combination, threaten vision and are the cause of so-called river blindness in Africa.

3 Control is being achieved in two ways. First, the breeding grounds of the *Simulium* flies are localized and so amenable to insecticide treatment. The insecticide may be applied on the ground or, in more remote areas, from the air. Second, cases or even whole populations in endemic areas may be treated with ivermectin. This reduces the number of persons with microfilariae in their skin and so reduces the risk of blackfly becoming infected and transmitting infection. With a combination of these approaches, onchocerciasis has been abolished from

some areas. However, continued vigilance is necessary to prevent re-establishment of the disease in these areas.

4 In cases, such as this one, where no microfilariae are detected in the skin snips, the diagnosis can be confirmed by the Mazzotti reaction. This is a local erythematous or urticarial reaction in the skin after a very small oral dose of DEC. It is essential that a Mazzotti test is only performed if skin snips are negative, and is supervised in hospital.

References

Goa KL, McTavish D & Clissold SP (1991) Ivermectin. A review of its antifilarial activity, pharmokinetic properties and clinical efficacy in onchocerciasis. *Drugs* **42**, 640–658.

Greene BM (1992) Modern medicine versus an ancient scourge: progress towards control of onchocerciasis. *J. Infect. Dis.* **166**, 15–21.

79 A 23-year-old student returned from a 3-week holiday in Nepal with diarrhoea, flatulence and abdominal bloating. This persisted for 4 weeks after her return. She was afebrile and had lost no weight. Her general practitioner sent a stool sample to the laboratory, where the organisms shown in Fig. 79.1 were seen. The doctor prescribed a 3 day course of metronidazole and the symptoms resolved. Two weeks later her symptoms had recurred.

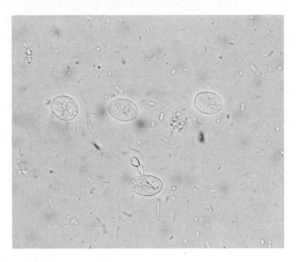

Fig. 79.1

Questions
1 What are the organisms seen in Fig. 79.1?
2 What is the site of infection?
3 What is the geographical distribution of this parasite?
4 How is it transmitted?
5 Why might the symptoms have recurred?

Answers 79

Answers

79

1 Cysts of *Giardia lamblia*. This is the stage of the parasite seen in faeces. It is protected from the environment by a thick wall and is infectious as soon as passed.

2 The active stage (trophozoite) lives in the small bowel where it attaches to the intestinal epithelium. In some people infection is asymptomatic, but it may result in a self-limiting diarrhoeal illness or even frank intestinal malabsorption. Occasionally, patients are seen with no cysts in the stools, but with an illness that resembles giardiasis. In these the trophozoites may be detected in jejunal aspirates, biopsies or string tests. This last involves swallowing a weighted string (Enterotest, HDC Corporation, San José, California, USA), the top end of which is fastened to the face. After a few hours the string is withdrawn and the jejunal juice milked from it and examined for trophozoites. The same technique can be used to detect *Strongyloides* larvae. Patients with malabsorption due to giardiasis may show a serological response to *Giardia* antigens which can be used diagnostically.

3 *Giardia* has a worldwide distribution. It does not require a warm climate for transmission and is endemic in the UK.

4 It is transmitted by the faecal–oral route. The cysts are small, resistant to chlorination and persist for weeks, and water-borne outbreaks have occurred. There is discussion about the role of animal reservoirs in giardiasis. Many mammals are infected with parasites which are morphologically similar to human isolates of G. *lamblia*, though they may differ biochemically and in their host-specificity. It is likely that in developed countries most giardiasis is acquired from human sources.

5 There are three main reasons why the infection may have recurred. First, metronidazole can occasionally result in side-effects of nausea and dizziness, so patients may not comply with treatment. This can be avoided by using single-dose treatment with a related agent, tinidazole. Second, resistance to imidazoles is recognized in *Giardia* and may account for treatment failure. Finally, immunodeficiency or other bowel pathology may prevent eradication. One specific association with persistent or recurrent giardiasis is immunoglobulin A (IgA) deficiency. In cases which do not respond to therapy, these causes should always be sought.

79 Reference

Hill DR (1990) *Giardia lamblia*. In: *Principles and Practice of Infectious Diseases*, 3rd edn (Mandell GL, Douglas RG & Bennett JE, eds), 2110–2115. Churchill Livingstone, New York.

A 28-year-old Venezuelan language student was seen in the accident and emergency department with grand mal convulsions. This was her first fit and there was no family history of epilepsy. Her family were from a poor rural area and regularly ate undercooked meat, including pork. Initial investigations, including full blood count, urea and electrolytes and lumbar puncture, were all normal. She responded well to standard anticonvulsant therapy, but a magnetic resonance imaging (MRI) brain scan revealed the lesion seen in Fig. 80.1.

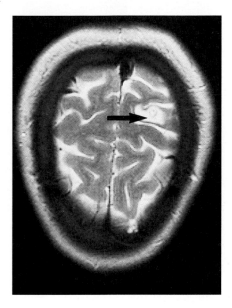

Fig. 80.1

80

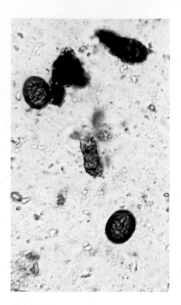

Fig. 80.2

Questions

1 What is the lesion seen in Fig. 80.1 and what is the diagnosis?
2 What are the bodies seen in Fig. 80.2 and what is their role in transmission?
3 Where else might the lesions be seen?
4 How might you confirm the diagnosis?
5 What treatment would you offer the patient?

Answers

1 This lesion is a cerebral cysticercus. This is the tissue stage of the pork tapeworm, *Taenia solium*. When the central nervous system is affected the condition is termed neurocysticercosis. It often presents with fits and in some parts of the world is the commonest cause of epilepsy.

2 These are Tania eggs; note the hooklets just visible inside. In uncomplicated infection the adult tapeworm is attached to the wall of the small intestine by its scolex. Segments grow out from this, maturing as they do so and filling with eggs. The end result is a flattened worm 2–7 metres long lying in the bowel lumen. The most distal segments break off when mature and are shed in the faeces. The eggs may be released in the bowel or when the segments rupture in the environment.

    The normal life cycle is for the eggs to be consumed by foraging pigs, to hatch in the gut and invade the blood, then to settle and produce cysticerci in the pigs tissues, particularly muscle. If infected pork is consumed by humans without proper cooking, the cysticerci evaginate in the small intestine where they attach to the bowel wall and grow into adult tapeworms, completing the cycle. Humans may also accidentally consume tapeworm eggs either from a contaminated environment or by the faecal–oral route. If this happens then the pig stage of the life cycle is followed and cysticerci are produced in the tissues. In the case described here the patient's consumption of undercooked pork was not what caused her infection. Where such dietary practices are prevalent, pork tapeworms are common and the risk of ingesting their eggs is increased.

3 Cysticerci can occur anywhere in the central nervous system. The presentation may be with hydrocephalus or meningitis, paralysis due to spinal cysticerci or visual symptoms due to ocular cysticerci. Most cysticerci are found in muscle and are usually asymptomatic. These are often calcified and noted as incidental findings on X-rays ordered for other purposes.

4 Confirmation of the diagnosis may be difficult. The finding of other cysticerci in X-rays of other tissues, such as thigh muscles, adds weight to the diagnosis. Cysticercosis elicits an immune response and serology may be valuable, as this is not usually positive in simple intestinal tapeworm infection. As with most serological tests, there are problems with cross-reactions (particularly with hydatid disease) and a pro-

80   portion of patients show no response. A recently developed technique, enzyme immunotransfer blotting (EITB) is reported to be more sensitive and specific than other serological tests, but it is not yet widely available.

5 Therapy is with either praziquantel or with albendazole, which kill the cysticerci, and steroids which prevent inflammatory reactions in the brain and worsening of symptoms. Standard anticonvulsant therapy is often also necessary.

Reference

Garcia HH, Martinez M, Gilman R, *et al.* (1991) Diagnosis of cysticercosis in endemic regions. *Lancet* **338**, 549–551.

Appendixes

Antibiotics

Antibiotics arranged in chemically or functionally similar grouping according to their principal site of action

Quinolones

nalidixic acid

narfloxacin
ciprofloxacin
ofloxacin
enoxacin
lomofloxacin
perfloxacin

Rifamycins
rifampicin
rifabutin

Cyclic peptides
bacitracin
polymyxin

Novobiocin

Phosphonate
fosmidomycin
fosfomycin

Glycopeptides
vancomycin
teichoplanin

Nitrofurans
nitrofurazone
nitrofurantoin

3rd generation broad
spectrum cephalosporins
cefotaxime
cefoperazone
cefsulodin
ceftizoxime
ceftrioxone
cefmenoxine
cefpirone

cephalosporins

cephamycins
cefoxitin
cefmetazole

cephalexin
cephradine
cefadroxil
cefaclor
cefuroxime

Nitroimidazoles
metronidazole
ornidazole
tinidazole

Sulphonamides
sulphadiazine
sulphamethoxazole
sulfadoxime
Trimethoprim

DNA

Cytoplasmic membrane

β-lactams

carbapenems
imipenem
meropenem

monobactams
aztreonam

50S binding
**Chloramphenicol
Fusidin
Clindamycin
Macrolides**

erythromycin
roxithromycin
clarithromycin
flurithromycin

azithromycin

Metabolism

tRNA binding
**Nananoic acid
Streptogramins**

30S binding
Aminoglycosides

neomycin spectinomycin kanamycin
gentamicin
tobramycin
netilmycin
amikacin

Tetracyclines
oxytetracycline
doxycycline
minocycline

Ribosomes

ureido and
aminobenzyl penicillin
ampicillin
amoxycillin

azlocillin
piperacillin

penicillins

isoxazole penicillins
oxacillin
cloxacillin
flucloxacillin
naficillin

benzylpenicillin
phenoxymethyl penicillin

MICROSCOPY

Gram stain
A general stain:
  Gram positive—blue/black
  Gram negative—red

Ziehl–Neelsen (ZN)
For mycobacteria:
  ZN positive—red
  Other bacteria—green

Dark ground microscopy
For *Treponema pallidum* and
Leptospira
the optics of the microscope
are adjusted so that the
object is bright against a
black background

Indian ink negative stain
To demonstrate presence
of capsule: used for
Cryptococcus in cerebrospinal fluid
(CSF)

Methenamine silver stain
For *Pneumocystis* and fungi

Immunofluorescent stains
Fluorescene labelled specific
antibodies used directly on
specimens, for example:
  Legionella
  Chlamydia
  T. pallidum

CULTURE

Aerobic
For most organisms

Anaerobic
For example for:
  Clostridia
  Bacteroides

Microaerobic
Campylobacter

NON-SELECTIVE MEDIA

Blood agar

Chocolate agar
Blood agar in which the erythrocytes
have been lysed, for example,
heat:
  used for *Haemophilus*
    Neisseria

SELECTIVE/DIFFERENTIAL MEDIA

For example:

CLED (cysteine lactose electrolyte-deficient)
Contains lactose and can differenti-
ate lactose fermenting (e.g.
Escherichia coli)
from non-lactose-fermenting
(e.g. *Pseudomonas*) bacteria.
Also inhibits swarming of *Proteus*
used for urine or wound swabs

DCA (deoxycholate citrate agar)
Contains lactose and can differentiate lactose fermenting (e.g. *E. coli*)
from non-lactose-fermenting
(e.g. *Salmonella*, *Shigella*)
bacteria; used for faeces

Skirrow medium
A blood-agar-based medium
containing antibiotics used to isolate
Campylobacter from faeces

Thayer–Martin medium
An enriched blood-agar-based
medium containing antibiotics used
to isolate *Neisseria gonorrhoeae*

Sabourauds medium
Used to culture fungi

Lowenstein–Jensen medium
Used to culture mycobacteria

SEROLOGY

ANTIGEN DETECTION

For example:

Latex particles (latex
agglutination) or
Staphylococcus aureus
(co-agglutination)
Coated with specific antibody
used to detect the presence
of antigen in clinical samples,
for example:
  Streptococcus pneumoniae
  H. influenzae
  N. meningitidis
  Cryptococcus neoformans in CSF

Bacterial Diagnosis

SEROLOGY

ANTIBODY DETECTION

Bacterial agglutination:
Killed suspension of bacteria used to detect specific antibodies in sera for diagnosis of, for example:
  Brucella
  Leptospira
  Legionella

Particle agglutination
For example: carbon, latex gelatin particles coated with antigen used to detect specific antibodies for diagnosis of
  syphilis (rapid plasma reagin test)
  S. pyogenes antibodies (anti-streptolysin O (ASO))
  Mycoplasma

Haemagglutination
Erythrocytes coated with antigen used to detect specific antibodies, for example:
  T. pallidum haemagglutination (TPHA)

Complement fixation test
For example, for diagnosing
  Q fever (*Coxiella burnetii*) and psittacosis (*Chlamydia psittaci*)

Enzyme-linked immunosorbent assay (ELISA)
Used for serological diagnosis of many infections, for example:
  Helicobacter pylori infection
  Lyme disease
  Clostridium difficile

Immunofluorescent antibody detection
For example, for syphilis—FTA (fluorescent *T. pallidum* antibody test)

MOLECULAR BIOLOGY

In-situ hybridization
The use of labelled DNA probes to detect the presence of pathogens, for example, enterotoxogenic *E. coli* in faeces

Polymerase chain reaction
Increasingly used method of detecting the presense of pathogens in clinical specimens, for example:
  Mycobacterium tuberculosis
  Pneumocystis carinii
  Mycoplasma pneumoniae
  Chlamydia trachomatis
  Legionella pneumophila

MISCELLANEOUS

Gas–liquid chromatography (GLC)
Used to detect volatile fatty acids in pus as a mark of the presence of anaerobic bacteria

Skin tests
For example, the Mantoux text

Cytopathic effect
Used to detect the presence of *C. difficile* toxin in faeces

Limulus endotoxin assay
Used to detect the presence of endotoxin in, for example, sera.

METHODS: A SUMMARY

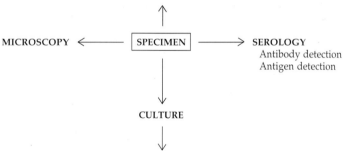

MOLECULAR BIOLOGY

MICROSCOPY ← SPECIMEN → SEROLOGY
Antibody detection
Antigen detection

↓

CULTURE

↓

Bacteriological **identification** of isolate by, for example, biochemical tests

↓

Sensitivity of isolate to antibiotics and typing (if appropriate):
  molecular biological methods, for example, ribotyping
  serotyping
  biotyping
  phage typing

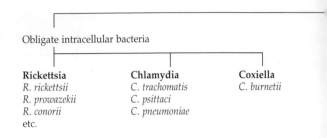

Obligate intracellular bacteria

Rickettsia	**Chlamydia**	**Coxiella**
R. rickettsii	*C. trachomatis*	*C. burnetii*
R. prowazekii	*C. psittaci*	
R. conorii	*C. pneumoniae*	
etc.		

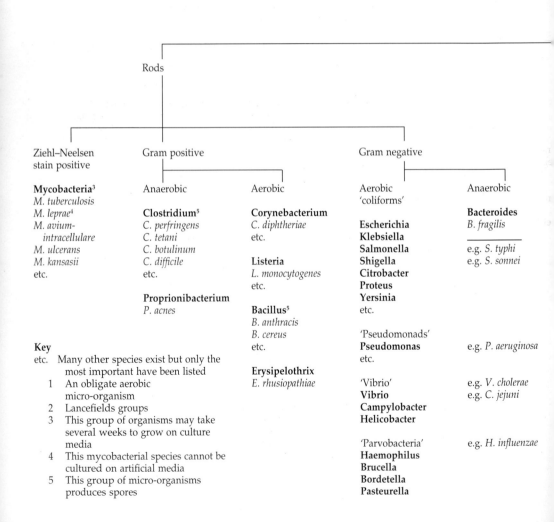

Rods

Ziehl–Neelsen stain positive	Gram positive		Gram negative	
	Anaerobic	Aerobic	Aerobic 'coliforms'	Anaerobic
Mycobacteria³		**Corynebacterium**		**Bacteroides**
M. tuberculosis	**Clostridium⁵**	*C. diphtheriae*	**Escherichia**	*B. fragilis*
M. leprae⁴	*C. perfringens*	etc.	**Klebsiella**	
M. avium-intracellulare	*C. tetani*		**Salmonella**	e.g. *S. typhi*
M. ulcerans	*C. botulinum*	**Listeria**	**Shigella**	e.g. *S. sonnei*
M. kansasii	*C. difficile*	*L. monocytogenes*	**Citrobacter**	
etc.	etc.	etc.	**Proteus**	
			Yersinia	
	Proprionibacterium		etc.	
	P. acnes	**Bacillus⁵**		
		B. anthracis	'Pseudomonads'	
		B. cereus	**Pseudomonas**	e.g. *P. aeruginosa*
		etc.	etc.	
		Erysipelothrix	'Vibrio'	e.g. *V. cholerae*
		E. rhusiopathiae	**Vibrio**	e.g. *C. jejuni*
			Campylobacter	
			Helicobacter	
			'Parvobacteria'	e.g. *H. influenzae*
			Haemophilus	
			Brucella	
			Bordetella	
			Pasteurella	

Key

etc. Many other species exist but only the most important have been listed
1 An obligate aerobic micro-organism
2 Lancefields groups
3 This group of organisms may take several weeks to grow on culture media
4 This mycobacterial species cannot be cultured on artificial media
5 This group of micro-organisms produces spores

of Bacteria

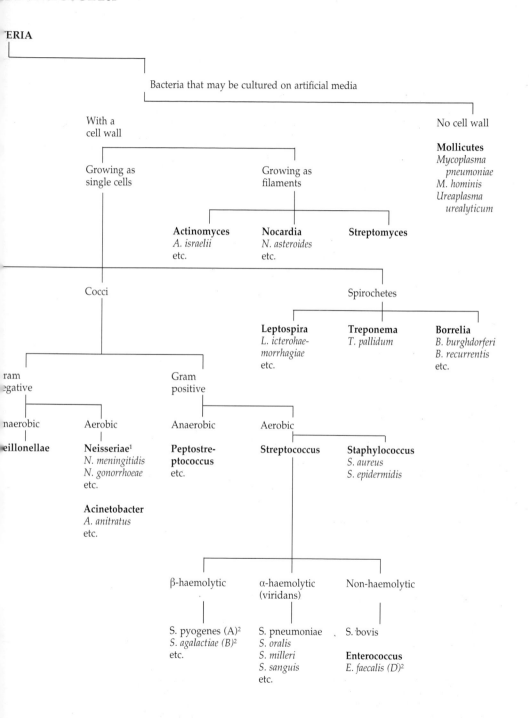

ERIA

Bacteria that may be cultured on artificial media

With a
cell wall

No cell wall

Mollicutes
*Mycoplasma
  pneumoniae*
M. hominis
*Ureaplasma
  urealyticum*

Growing as
single cells

Growing as
filaments

Actinomyces
A. israelii
etc.

Nocardia
N. asteroides
etc.

Streptomyces

Cocci

Spirochetes

Leptospira
*L. icterohae-
morrhagiae*
etc.

Treponema
T. pallidum

Borrelia
B. burghdorferi
B. recurrentis
etc.

ram
egative

Gram
positive

naerobic

Aerobic

Anaerobic

Aerobic

eillonellae

Neisseriae[1]
N. meningitidis
N. gonorrhoeae
etc.

Acinetobacter
A. anitratus
etc.

**Peptostre-
ptococcus**
etc.

Streptococcus

Staphylococcus
S. aureus
S. epidermidis

β-haemolytic

α-haemolytic
(viridans)

Non-haemolytic

S. pyogenes (A)[2]
S. agalactiae (B)[2]
etc.

S. pneumoniae
S. oralis
S. milleri
S. sanguis
etc.

S. bovis

Enterococcus
E. faecalis (D)[2]